Vagus Stimulation

UNLEASH THE FULL POTENTIAL OF VAGUS NERVE
STIMULATION THROUGH SPECIFIC EXERCISES,
ELIMINATE ANXIETY AND DEPRESSION,
AND ACHIEVE MAXIMUM WELL-BEING

Suzanne Illingworth

Table of Contents

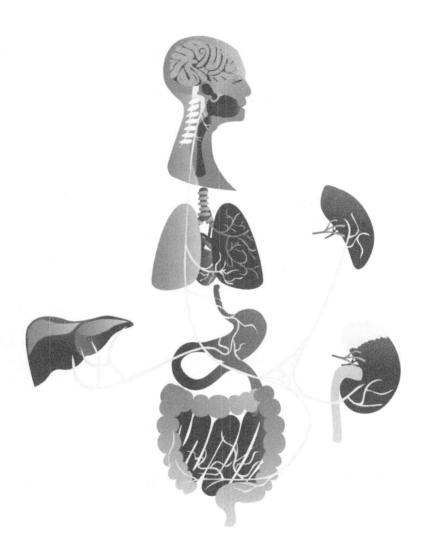

Introduction

If you are struggling with an autoimmune disease, a weakened immune system, or vagus nerve damage, expanding your knowledge about the functions of the vagus nerve and the benefits you might gain from its stimulation could be a valuable aid for you. By stimulating and improving the state of tension in the vagus nerve, you can reduce symptoms and improve your overall well-being. However, it may take some time for the effects to take hold; with patience, small lifestyle changes can make a big difference.

The vagus nerve is critical to maintaining your well-being because it affects so many different parts of your body. As a part of the nervous system, it keeps your heart beating, lungs breathing, and the digestive system working. It even plays a role in regulating hormones and your voice. By keeping your vagus nerve healthy and functioning correctly, you can influence and ensure the health of your entire body.

In order for your organs to function properly and maintain optimal health, it's essential to have a balanced state in your body. This balance is controlled by the sympathetic and parasympathetic nervous systems, which prepare your body to fight threats and keep it rested and relaxed, respectively. Achieving this balance creates an ideal environment for your body to activate its natural self-healing mechanisms and maintain good health.

The vagus nerve is also essential for achieving balance in the body. As the longest cranial nerve, it plays a vital role in transmitting messages between the organs and the brain. It ensures that essential physiological processes like blood supply to the heart muscle and heart rate and blood pressure regulation function smoothly. Persistent sympathetic responses can lead to chronic inflammation and autoimmune diseases without proper vagal activity.

However, by inhibiting the effects of sympathetic responses, the vagus nerve creates an optimal environment for the body's natural self-healing mechanisms to maintain and renew cells, thus promoting physical and mental well-being. By learning how to activate and stimulate the vagus nerve, we can tap into our body's natural self-healing powers to prevent diseases, manage mental disorders, and reduce the severity of chronic illnesses.

In the upcoming chapters, we will explore the body's remarkable self-healing abilities and how to activate them through the vagus nerve. As the largest cranial nerve, the vagus nerve is found throughout the body, controlling both motor and sensory functions of various organs and keeping the body in balance by regulating the fight or flight responses of the sympathetic nervous system.

Although the vagus nerve is naturally active, certain factors like age and stress can inhibit its activity, leading to decreased vagal tone. Therefore, learning to activate and stimulate the vagus nerve is crucial to taking advantage of its self-healing powers, preventing certain diseases, and treating chronic inflammation and related conditions like rheumatoid arthritis.

By mastering the powers of the largest cranial nerve, you can significantly improve your health and create a natural pathway for your body to heal and repair itself. Understanding the workings of the body and how to keep essential elements like the vagus nerve constantly stimulated and active is vital to maintaining good health.

So let's get started and explore how to harness the powers of the vagus nerve for optimal health and well-being.

Chapter 1 Detailed explanation of the vagus nerve: anatomy and functions

The vagus nerve

The vagus nerve, also known as the "wandering nerve," is a dynamic duo of cranial nerves that sprout from the brain stem and spread throughout the body like curious vagabonds. This nerve earns its name because of its extensive reach, stretching through the face, neck, torso, and abdomen, influencing and supplying many different body areas. This nerve is unique because it is "sensorimotor," which means it has the unique ability to communicate with both the brain and the body. It can send signals and sensory data to the brain while also receiving commands from the brain to control the body's movements. Essentially, the vagus nerve not only has to make sense, but it also has to get things moving!

This nerve is crucial for regulating emotions, dealing with stress, and interacting with others. It plays a vital role in the parasympathetic nervous system, which controls critical bodily functions such as metabolism, immune response, posture regulation, and heart rate. In fact, activating the vagus nerve may even be a promising therapy for drug-resistant anxiety, post-traumatic stress disorder, and inflammatory bowel disease.

The vagus nerve is like a superhero, regulating the autonomic nervous system and enabling the natural fear response of the human body. It allows you to react instinctively and make quick decisions in life-or-death situations without wasting precious time thinking about them. In addition, the nerve interacts with crucial body parts, such as the heart, lungs, and digestive tract, making it essential for regulating those functions.

So, if you're grateful for your heart beating, lungs breathing, and digestion doing its job, don't forget to thank the vagus nerve! This wandering nerve keeps your body in check and allows you to survive and thrive.

The functions of the vagus nerve

The vagus nerve is a true multitasker - it's involved in various bodily functions, but at its core, it's a sensory receptor that carries information from the body to the brain. So this nerve is responsible for keeping the body in check by constantly adapting to sensory input. And it has a lot to do with it!

The vagus nerve has four main functions, each receiving sensory input from different body parts. These functions are as follows:

Sensory input: The vagus nerve receives information from the heart, lungs, throat, and abdomen.

Taste input: It also has a hand in creating the sensation of taste.

Motor: The vagus nerve is responsible for movement within the muscles necessary for swallowing and speaking.

Parasympathetic nervous system: This nerve regulates digestion, breathing, and heart rate.

But wait, there's more! These four functions can be broken down into seven distinct tasks, which allow the vagus nerve to regulate even more of the body. Here are those functions:

1. Control of the sympathetic nervous system: The vagus nerve regulates alertness, the circulatory system, and breathing. This means the brain can directly control the nervous system, producing high energy and attention.
2. Regulation of the parasympathetic nervous system: On the other hand, this system reduces alertness and activates the state of rest and digestion.
3. Facilitation of communication between the brain and the gut: The vagus nerve creates a pathway for signals to travel from the gut and digestive system to the brain.
4. Enabling and triggering relaxation: The vagus nerve can cause the diaphragm to slow down, resulting in deeper breathing and further relaxation.
5. Anti-inflammatory: This nerve can have an anti-inflammatory effect, leading to a decrease in inflammation levels.

6. Regulation of heart rate and blood pressure: The vagus nerve regulates heart rate and blood pressure. When it's not functioning properly, it can lead to issues such as unconsciousness or a rise in blood pressure.

7. Anxiety regulation: Because the vagus nerve regulates the sympathetic and parasympathetic nervous systems, it can signal the body when it's time to relax and handle anxiety.

In short, the vagus nerve is an absolute superstar when it comes to keeping the body in check. Whether anxious or relaxed, hungry or complete, the vagus nerve ensures your body functions at its best.

The Basic Anatomy of the Vagus

The vagus nerve (also known as the 10th cranial nerve, CN X) is a long nerve that runs from the brain tube to the neck, chest, and up to abdomen. It supplies the heart, major blood vessels, respiratory system, kidneys, esophagus, stomach, and intestines when both motor and sensory information is present. Although there are two vagus nerves, the left and right, doctors refer to them collectively as the "vagus nerve." It is essential for maintaining a healthy gastrointestinal tract and controlling the heart rate. The vagus nerves also carry sensory information from the internal organs to the brain.

The "vagus nerve" is the most important parasympathetic nerve in the body. It distributes parasympathetic fibers to all body organs, including major organs such as the heart and lungs. It is the main pathway for transmitting information between the brain and other body organs and tissues. Thus, it enables the brain to monitor the functions of various body organs and systems.

Structurally, the vagus nerve runs from the medulla oblongata through the jugular foramen to the inferior cerebellar peduncle. It then runs in the carotid sheath between the internal jugular vein and the internal carotid artery before descending from the thorax and neck into the abdomen. The vagus nerve contributes to the supply of the viscera, which extends down to the colon.

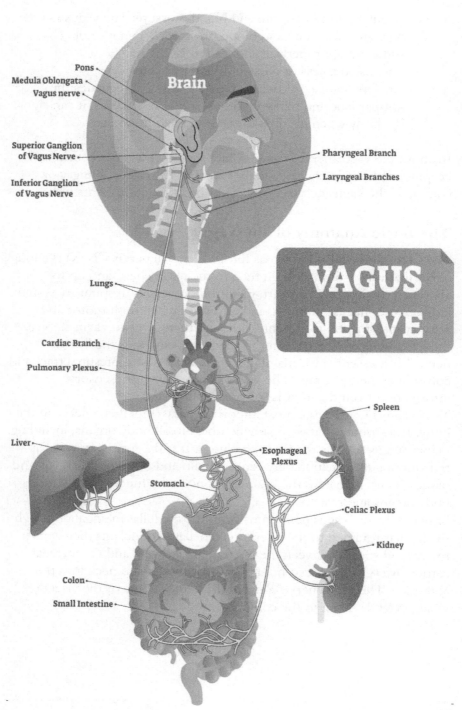

The vagus nerve contains up to 90 % of the afferent nerves that transmit sensory information about the condition of various body organs to the central nervous system. The right and left vagus nerves emerge from the cranial vault, cross the jugular foramina and enter the carotid sheath between the carotid arteries. They then connect to the common carotid artery via the posterolateral artery. The cell bodies of the visceral afferent fibers of the vagus nerve are located bilaterally in its inferior ganglion.

The right vagus nerve stimulates the right recurrent laryngeal nerve, which wraps around the right subclavian artery. It then ascends to the throat and crosses both the esophagus and trachea. The right vagus nerve then crosses the right subclavian artery and returns to the superior vena cava. It then descends behind the right main bronchus and spreads across the esophageal, cardiac, and pulmonary plexus. Finally, in the lower esophagus, it forms the posterior vagal trunk and then passes through the diaphragm via the esophageal hiatus.

Meanwhile, the left vagus nerve descends the aortic arch after passing through the chest between the left common carotid artery and the left subclavian artery. It ascends between the esophagus and trachea by lifting the left recurrent laryngeal nerve and hooks around the aortic arch on the left side of the ligamentum arteriosum. The left vagus arises from the thoracic, cardiac branches, which split into the pulmonary plexus and descend to the esophageal plexus. Finally, it enters the abdomen as the anterior vagus trunk through the esophageal hiatus of the diaphragm.

The vagus nerve emerges from the brain's medulla and exits the skull through the foramen jugular located at its base. Meanwhile, its auricular branch exits within the skull to provide sensory feedback to the auditory canal and pinna. Finally, traversing via the carotid sheath, the vagus nerve makes its way from the head to the neck. In the neck, the vagus nerve runs with the jugular vein and the inferior carotid artery to the base of the neck, where the right and left vagus nerves branch into two separate cords. The right vagus nerve enters the thorax via the anterior subclavian artery and the posterior sternoclavicular joint. The left vagus nerve, on the other hand, enters the thorax and runs behind the sternoclavicular joint and between the carotid artery and the left subclavian artery.

In the neck, the vagus nerve branches into:

Superior laryngeal nerve: This nerve consists of inner and outer branches. The external branch of the laryngeal nerve provides sensory innervation to the larynx through the cricothyroid muscle. The internal laryngeal nerve innervates the laryngopharynx.

The pharyngeal branch: The nerve that motorically innervates the soft palate and pharynx muscles.

Recurrent laryngeal nerve: This nerve runs from the right subclavian artery to the larynx and innervates the larynx muscles.

When the vagus nerve reaches the chest, it divides into the posterior and anterior vagus trunks. The left vagus nerve forms the anterior vagus trunk, while the right vagus nerve forms the rear vagus trunk. The esophageal plexus, created by these vagus trunks, innervates the smooth muscles of the esophagus.

The branches, originating in the thorax, innervate the heart muscles and regulate the heart rate. The left laryngeal recurrent nerve innervates most of the laryngeal muscles. The vagal trunks run from the thorax into the abdomen via an opening in the diaphragm called the esophageal hiatus.

The vagal trunks divide into several branches in the abdominal cavity and supply the small and large intestines, the stomach, and the esophagus.

The vagus nerve transmits various signals from the digestive system and organs to the brain and vice versa.

The vagus nerve exits the bulb through the groove between the olive and the inferior structural pedicle and goes the os jugular through the middle compartment of the jugular opening. The vagus nerve innervates most of the throat muscles and the vocal organ responsible for swallowing and vocalization in the throat. In addition, it provides the primary parasympathetic supply to the heart and stimulates a reduction in velocity in the chest.

Let's make this description of the vagus nerve a bit more fun and easy to understand!

Have you ever wondered how your body knows when to digest your food? Or how do you automatically swallow when you take a big gulp of water? Well, you can thank the mighty vagus nerve for that!

The vagus nerve is like an orchestra conductor, controlling the movements of the muscles and organs in your digestive system. It comprises preganglionic neurons (fancy word for nerve cells) that connect to your intestine and tells it when to contract and release essential juices to break down your food.

But that's not all! The vagus nerve also has a celiac branch that connects the different parts of your intestine. It's like a superhighway for messages telling your body what to do.

And if that wasn't impressive enough, it also has sensors throughout your body that can detect changes in pressure, chemicals, and even electricity. These sensors help your body know when it's time to cough, sneeze, or swallow, and they send signals to your brain to make it all happen.

These messages are transmitted through the vagus nerve and relayed to different parts of your brain, including the locus coeruleus, the rostral ventrolateral medulla, and the ganglion. It's like a giant communication network, all thanks to the mighty vagus nerve!

So next time you enjoy a delicious meal or feel the urge to sneeze, take a moment to thank your fantastic vagus nerve for making it all possible.

Chapter 2: The Polyvagal Theory

In 1994, Dr. Stephen Porges of the University of Illinois proposed the polyvagal theory for the first time.

The polyvagal theory explains three different components of our sensory system and their reactions to stressful situations.

Understanding these three sections helps us understand why and how we react to high-pressure levels. In addition, it is a compelling explanation of how our body deals with intense pressure and how we can reduce the severity of the injury with different treatments.

This theory states that the nerve has a distinct hierarchical model with three subdivisions. These are:

The dorsal vagal system

The dorsal vagus nerve is a large nerve that runs from the brain through the spine to the lungs, heart, and stomach. It is present in all animals and plays a role in sleep and relaxation:

- Heartbeat control
- Breathing control
- Helps with digestion.

We have seen how animals freeze in danger. Imagine encountering a deer in your car at night. It may become so frightened that it freezes on the road and becomes immobile while staring into the headlights. Possums have also been observed to "freeze" when in danger, then move again when they feel safe. But have you ever wondered how this happens? After all, animals are not intelligent enough to "play dead," are they?

As mentioned earlier, the autonomic nervous system performs sympathetic and parasympathetic functions. When we are in danger or under stress, our sympathetic nervous system kicks in to facilitate the fight or flight response we use to protect ourselves. We try to cope with stress or dangerous circumstances by fighting or fleeing.

We have two options when we encounter a vicious dog: pick up a stick and fight it or run away. However, when our fight or flight mechanisms fail to cope with the stress, the sympathetic nervous system can become so overstimulated that our body can no longer cope. Once this happens, the parasympathetic nervous system reacts so strongly to the overstimulation of the sympathetic nervous system that it puts the body into a "frozen" state.

Immobilization, dissociation, emotional distance, or the inability to think clearly are all symptoms of this "freeze" state. This state can be short-lived, as in the case of the possum, and end as soon as the threat has passed, or it can last for a more extended period of time or even indefinitely.

Because it is present in almost all vertebrate species, the dorsal branch is called the older vagus nerve. While the ventral branch causes a state of engagement, the dorsal branch is a little more complex. Its primary function is to induce a state of shutdown.

This immobilization is divided into two types: Immobilization with and without fear. When our fight-flight response is ineffective, we simply give up and freeze. This reaction is caused by fear taking complete control of us. On the other hand, when wholly relaxed and the dorsal branch is working with the ventral circulation, we are immobilized without fear. Think of this as choosing to be intimate with someone to build a stronger bond.

Given the importance that every living thing's biological system places on survival, one might ask why it should be an excellent strategy to shut it down or immobilize it. Isn't that a death sentence for any living thing? Immobilization can also be interpreted as slowing down. Hibernation, for example, is an activity involving dorsal circulation. To survive the harsh winter conditions, a bear in hibernation uses a survival mechanism that involves lowering its body temperature and breathing. Reptiles go one step further by almost completely freezing and shutting down their body functions. For this reason, snakes can survive for long periods without feeding. Mice are another example of how immobilization facilitates survival.

When a mouse is confronted with a predator like a goshawk, which can detect and hunt scurrying mice from miles above, it shuts down completely, holds its breath, and remains motionless in front of the goshawk. It is, therefore, more difficult for the bird of prey to detect telltale movements of the mouse. When the threat is over, the mouse returns to its routine.

Of course, this can backfire. Deer and mice often freeze in the face of a predator or threat. The expression "deer in headlights" aptly describes a fear-induced shutdown. This results from an extreme shutdown at a pace that is clearly too fast for the animal to process what is going on. Chronic activation of the dorsal circuit is responsible for the shutdown. In other words, look at how a depressed or anxious person behaves. First, they withdraw from the environment because they cannot process everything happening in the world. Remaining in this state for a more extended period leads to even higher levels of depression and anxiety.

I want to emphasize that when I use "depression," I refer to the feeling, not the medical diagnosis. This is not to say that a medical diagnosis of depression is different. Instead, the initial feeling and the diagnosis simply reflect different levels of activity of the dorsal branch, the latter reflecting far greater activity.

Trauma or a sudden death threat can cause us to shut down entirely as the survival mechanism kicks in. Of course, the reasons for this mechanism to kick in may not be justified. Still, again, this only happens when events external to us overwhelm our brain's processing capacity to figure out what is going on. In this case, the dorsal branch is reflexively activated, and we often put ourselves in even greater danger. People who can function well come out of this state as soon as the danger has passed, but chronic activation of the dorsal circuit means that people remain in this state much longer than necessary.

The sympathetic system

As we learned in the previous chapter, our sympathetic nervous system is part of the autonomic nervous system that enables the body to respond to stimuli. This system controls our fight and flight responses and acts on the following body organs:

- The heart - it increases the heart rate

- The lungs - increase breathing by dilating the bronchi
- The intestine - causes constriction of the gastrointestinal muscles and organs.
- Digestive tract - inhibits food movement along the tract (peristalsis).
- Blood vessels - it causes the blood vessels to dilate to increase blood flow
- The eye - it causes pupil dilation
- Sweat glands - it stimulates the secretion of sweat
- Kidney - it inhibits the secretion of renin
- Penis - it inhibits an erection

These effects prepare the body for action by increasing access to energy reserves, improving cardiac and respiratory functions, and enabling us to fight or flee from threats. These stress responses balance the relaxation effects of the parasympathetic nervous system. The sympathetic and parasympathetic systems work closely together to create balance in the function of the internal body organs and achieve a homeostatic state in the body.

The ventral vagus system

According to the Polyvagal theory, the third division of the vagus nerve is the parasympathetic system of social engagement, which is attributed to the ventral vagus nerve. This nerve is found in mammals that care for their offspring and typically lead to the facial muscles.

The ventral vagus system is myelinated to increase and control reaction speed. Because it influences our adaptive and prosocial behavior, this nerve is also known as the "intelligent vagus." It has been shown that people with a higher vagus tone are better able to engage socially and adapt more flexibly to different social situations.

The ventral vagus system inhibits sympathetic stimulation of the heart, which means that when it is active, it has a calming effect that can be conducive to social engagement. For example, suppose you are anxious or under emotional stress. In that case, you are less likely to want to socialize or form an emotional bond with others because you are not receptive to social interaction. The ventral vagus system creates a sense of calmness by counteracting and inhibiting sympathetic effects on our bodily organs, which tends to put us in a more positive mood and emotional state.

The ventral branch and the four cranial nerves it interacts with are responsible for calm social interaction. Physical health and the absence of danger or the fight or flight response are prerequisites for healthy social interaction. In such a state, we can relax and act with composure. The ventral branch coordinates the feeling of calm and other psychological conditions necessary for several socially essential functions to promote this state of well-being.

Bonding with our children, building friendships and relationships, working together, etc., all depend on regulation by the ventral branch. The ventral branch is often called the "younger" branch of the vagus nerve. This relates to how our species, like everything else, has evolved. The ventral circuit is unique to mammals and is not found in other vertebrate species. Whether such a circuit exists in birds is controversial but has not been definitively proven(Gehin, 2007). However, since mammals are more evolved than other vertebrates, it is assumed that the ventral circuit is evolutionarily younger.

When the fight or flight response kicks in, the ventral circuitry shuts down entirely, and we resort to less developed responses such as fight or flight. Withdrawal can be associated with depression and anxiety. These primitive reactions are often observed in creatures that lack this circuitry, although the flight is a very different phenomenon in humans and reptiles (Gehin, 2007).

Contrary to popular belief, the social engagement aspect of human interaction is equally responsible for our protection and other evolutionary responses. For example, we often think of making new friends or partners when we engage socially. However, we are unaware that a socially engaged attitude toward the world can protect us from many dangers.

We will inevitably trigger a conflict if we approach a potentially threatening situation with our fight-or-flight response. However, if we engage socially positively, the potential threat often defuses itself as the other person's social bonding need is also activated. People with healthy ventral circuits thus use their flight-and-fight response only as a last resort and therefore avoid shutting down their socially engaged side.

When the autonomic nervous system detects a threat, it switches from a highly developed and socially engaged response to one similar to a reptile. If this response is also insufficient, the brain shuts down and withdraws.

The Importance of the Polyvagal Theory

For professionals and lovers of pop-brain science, understanding polyvagal theory can be helpful: to understand injury and post-traumatic stress disorder (PTSD) and the movement of attack and withdrawal, to see how tremendous pressure leads to disconnection or shutdown, to recognize how to perceive non-verbal communication. We like to think of our feelings as ethereal, complex, and challenging to sort out and identify. In reality, feelings are reactions to an impulse (internal or external). Often they occur outside of our awareness, especially when we are out of tune with our enthusiastic inner life. Our fundamental desire to stay alive is more important to our body than our ability to think about staying alive. This is where the polyvagal theory comes in. The sensory system is constantly running out of sight, controlling our bodily capacities so that we can think about different things - like what kind of dessert we want or how to get a prestigious one. The entire sensory system works together with the mind and can take control of our passionate experience, regardless of whether we need it.

Chapter 3: How can vagus nerve stimulation help reduce anxiety and depression?

Every day more people are diagnosed with anxiety, depression, and other mental health problems. What is the cause of this increase in the number of people with mental health problems? What are our options to counteract it? As you might expect, the answer lies in the vagus nerve, as with many other health problems. It doesn't matter whether the issues are mental or physical; they are all influenced by the nervous system, which produces the hormones needed to control mood.

When it comes to anxiety and depression, most people turn to medication to counteract it. For doctors treating patients with mental illness, they are often the drug of choice. Medication can be effective, but what if there was a better way? Is there a way to avoid the side effects these drugs can cause? Many people have experienced relief by stimulating the vagus nerve. This is not some strange alternative medicine, but a scientifically based method that we want to examine how it works.

Anxieties and the vagus nerve

To understand the relationship between the vagus nerve and anxiety, we must first understand the action of the two components of the nervous system. Simply put, the sympathetic nervous system prepares the body for action. Producing hormones, such as adrenaline, only prepares the body for action. On the other hand, the parasympathetic nervous system only helps the body to enter a state of rest.

Anxiety only starts when a person gets into a stressful situation. When one gets into a stressful situation, the sympathetic nervous system switches to overdrive. If the stress continues and the body takes too long to shut down the activated physiological changes, the body can suffer greatly. For example, when the sympathetic nervous system is activated, the person cannot perform parasympathetic activities such as deep sleep. We all know that rest is vital for the body and that one is more likely to suffer without it.

When stress is prolonged, two pathways in the brain are activated simultaneously (the hypothalamic-pituitary-adrenal axis and brain-gut axis). Usually, the brain responds to stress (anxiety) by producing more of the corticotropin-releasing factor (CRF). The hormones travel from the hypothalamus to the pituitary glands, stimulating the production of other hormones called steroid hormones (ACTH). When ACTH is produced, it travels through the bloodstream to the adrenal glands, activating cortisol and adrenal induction. When the adrenal glands are activated, they act as an immune system, protecting the body from internal injuries caused by stress. If the stress is ongoing or chronic, the physiological changes in the body are likely to outweigh the body's ability to cope and function. Finally, the combination of stress and physical failure can have devastating consequences, such as depression. Many studies have linked depression to inflammatory responses in the brain. Since stress is a precursor to inflammation, it is crucial to find a way to manage stress before it becomes uncontrollable.

Chronic stress can also lead to increased glutamate production. When this neurotransmitter is produced in abundance, it is known to trigger migraines. Some research has also linked depression and anxiety to excessive glutamate production. Stress can also cause other psychological problems. For example, cortisol production can reduce the hippocampus volume, the part of the brain responsible for forming new memories. This explains why anxious people often forget further information.

The involvement of the vagus nerve in stress management can lead to complications. Since the vagus nerve cannot activate relaxation signals, the sympathetic nervous system maintains control, which can lead to insomnia, gastrointestinal problems, and shortness of breath, among other things.

The vagus nerve, as mentioned earlier, activates the parasympathetic nervous system to establish the body's state of rest and digestion. Conversely, a lack of activation of the vagus nerve allows the sympathetic nervous system to give free rein to the body and control it completely. This leads to an increase in stress hormones, which in turn causes inflammation that can affect the brain, among other things. However, the longer the sympathetic nervous system rules, the more stressed and anxious the body becomes, leading to higher levels of cortisol and glutamate, which continue to stress the body. This process explains how one feels depressed.

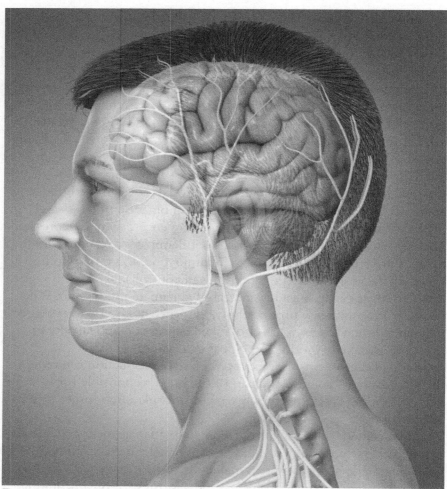

Because of its afferent status, the vagus nerve naturally sends impulses back to the brain to tell how the body feels. The longer the stress lasts, the less likely it is that the parasympathetic nervous system will be activated at all and the less likely it is that you will be able to overcome the anxiety at a later stage. You will have a hard time if you cannot get your vagus nerve going again and get it moving.

People who suffer from anxiety are more likely to worry than others. But this is no ordinary worry. It has the potential to negatively affect a person's life and cause them to give up activities they enjoy because they are overly stressed. Agitation occurs, which manifests itself in increased heart rate, sweating, and faster breathing. They can also get tired quickly and feel tense, irritable, restless, and need to move because they simply cannot sit still. Panic attacks are also common, and many people who suffer from anxiety cannot sleep for worry. How does this situation come about?

Previously, we learned about the fight-or-flight response, designed to protect us. This is dependent on the vagus nerve. The sympathetic nervous system causes your body to produce adrenaline, which gives you the boost you need to fight off or flee from enemies. Your sympathetic nervous system is activated when you are in a stressful situation, even if it is not dangerous. When the nervous system signals to the brain that you are in danger, various glands begin to produce hormones such as adrenaline and cortisol.

These two hormones suppress the immune system. As a result, the body is wholly geared towards fight or flight. That's why people who are frequently stressed or suffer from anxiety and panic attacks get sick more often than their peers.

In addition to these hormones, stress activates two different pathways in the nervous system. One of these is the brain-gut pathway, which can cause significant digestive problems. For example, when you are anxious and stressed, your intestines can spasm, and you can get diarrhea. This is because the nervous system causes your bowels to contract. Similarly, it can cause nausea and vomiting in the stomach. The sympathetic nervous system also makes the heart beat faster, constricts the blood vessels, and dilates the bronchioles so that all the energy and resources are focused on the areas of the body needed for fight or flight. The idea is to temporarily divert blood flow to the heart and muscles so you can survive whatever comes your way. That's fine when it's life and death when you're up against an assassin or a lion, but when it's just a matter of turning in a project late or worrying that you left the cooker on, it's too much of a good thing.

Anxiety symptoms are due to the vagus nerve, which can cause everything from palpitations and arrhythmias to hyperventilating. This is all due to the involvement of this part of the nervous system, and if nothing is done about it, the anxiety and its symptoms will persist for an extended period of time.

Anxiety disorders are becoming more common these days, and new drugs are constantly coming on the market to treat this overreaction of the sympathetic nervous system. However, it is possible to stimulate the vagus nerve, activate the parasympathetic system and reduce the effects of anxiety. This is an inexpensive, drug-free way to lower heart rate and blood pressure, but few people know how to use this technique.

Depression and the vagus nerve

Although most forms of depression can be treated with less invasive methods, the fact that vagus nerve stimulation can treat depression suggests that there is some connection. While it is unclear why vagus nerve stimulation can improve depression, particularly treatment-resistant depression, which has been challenging to treat in the past, it has been shown to be effective.

This is not surprising because the vagus nerve is responsible for maintaining the relaxed state in which humans can sleep. However, the sympathetic nervous system can take over if the vagus nerve cannot activate the parasympathetic nervous system to control the body. So it wreaks havoc on the body for too long. As with everything else, moderation is key - a certain amount of stress is beneficial and even motivating, but inflammation begins when the sympathetic nervous system dominates the mind.

This inflammation, in particular, can be linked to depression. It has been found that people who have elevated levels of inflammation can experience depressed moods. In addition, inflammation reduces serotonin levels in the brain, leading to mood regulation problems. Finally, depression is commonly treated with selective serotonin reuptake inhibitors (SSRIs), which increase serotonin levels in the brain to relieve symptoms.

The result is that a lack of vagus nerve stimulation overloads the sympathetic nervous system. This causes inflammatory reactions in the body, which in turn causes the body to have difficulty producing enough serotonin. The lack of serotonin is therefore associated with depressive symptoms.

Depression, like anxiety, can be a complex subject. Depression has only recently been classified as a mental illness, and only now is it beginning to be understood. Dealing with chronic depression can be challenging and even lead to self-harm and suicide. It can also manifest as bipolar disorder, where the person is depressed for a while before becoming manic. When a person is manic, they cannot sleep and seem highly energetic and hyper. They may have lots of ideas and want to be very creative. However, this is usually only the case temporarily.

Lack of interest in activities, hopelessness, weight loss or gain, changes in sleeping habits (too much or too little sleep), anger, irritability, tiredness and fatigue, poor decision-making as well as reckless behavior, difficulty concentrating and pain or aching body parts for no apparent reason are all symptoms of depression. Stomach and chest pains are widespread. In addition, stress leads to constant headaches and even toothache or earache in many people with depression. Although everyone occasionally experiences sadness, natural depression goes much deeper than that. It can manifest without any identifiable cause or trigger, and just because someone cannot pinpoint the reason behind their depression does not diminish the validity of their emotions. Instead, it is likely related to the nervous system affecting the person's thoughts or feelings.

Many factors play a role in the development of depression. Nearly 17% of Americans suffer from depression, which genetic factors, biological problems, environmental stress, inflammation, poor hormone regulation and nervous system dysfunction can cause. Determining which of these problems is the trustworthy source would be pointless, as they all contribute.

In the brain, the amino acid tryptophan contributes to the production of serotonin, the happiness hormone. If this amino acid is not present in the body in sufficient quantities, it can prevent proper hormone production and cause one to feel hopeless, sad, and depressed. In addition, an increase in inflammation in the brain or prolonged inflammation can lead to lower serotonin levels, which in turn can cause depression.

Stimulating the vagus nerve can help reduce inflammation in the body as the nerve tells the immune system that it can calm down a little. As a result, the inflammation in the body, including the brain, is reduced so normal functions can resume.

The vagus nerve's role in chronic depression may not be the best-researched nervous system area, but it dramatically impacts mental health. Therefore, it is essential to stimulate the vagus nerve and improve the vagal tone so that you can enjoy good mental health. However, this does not mean you should stop taking your medication if you are taking any. Instead, you should always discuss the best way to prevent your medicine with a doctor, as some can have serious side effects if stopped abruptly.

Chapter 4: What is the vagus nerve-based neuro-immune system?

The immune system

The immune system is the mechanism by which the body defends itself against disease or infection. It is made up of different types of white blood cells. Phagocytes are immune cells that attack bacteria or viruses that have invaded the body. Lymphocytes, another type of white blood cell, then document the structure of the virus or bacteria so that the body remembers the invaded pathogen and can prevent it from returning in the future. Both phagocytes and lymphocytes come in different shapes and sizes, and each is a specialized soldier for its area of responsibility - some are trained to provide general care, while others are more specialized. B lymphocytes, for example, go after targets that need to be defeated before signaling to the system that it needs help.

The immune system functions in different ways and generates three types of immunity. Humans can all have innate immunity, adaptive immunity, and passive immunity. Each of these forms works differently, but the result is that the body has some form of defense against disease. People with each form of immunity have a slightly different type of immunity with a somewhat different effect.

The human nervous and immune systems support our internal defense mechanisms. As humans, we are vulnerable to different types of attacks. Infections by disease-causing microorganisms such as bacteria or viruses are possible. A cold is almost always the result of a viral infection. Pneumonia, flu, sore throat, and bronchitis are all common illnesses caused by pathogenic infections.

The immune system operates by identifying and combating pathogens within the body, which implies that our capacity to resist and recuperate from infections is contingent upon the immune system's aptitude to recognize and eradicate the pathogen responsible for the illness. Pathogens are antigens from other organisms that invade our cells and disrupt normal cell function. Pathogens that invade the body include microorganisms such as bacteria, viruses, and fungi.

The immune system's task is to recognise and eliminate pathogens with the help of the cells that make it up, such as white blood cells, to restore cellular function. The immune system must be able to recognize its own cells and differentiate them from foreign or invading pathogens to function properly.

Inflammation is one of the mechanisms by which the immune system detects and fights infections caused by pathogens while healing itself. The immune system triggers an inflammatory response to help heal wounds, infections caused by pathogens, or tissue damage.

Inflammatory responses such as swelling after an injury, wound redness, or pus secretions indicate that the body is actively fighting the infection by sending white blood cells to the site of the condition. The healing of wounds, infections, and tissue damage would be impossible without inflammation.

Inflammation can occur when our sympathetic nervous system or immune system is overactive and attacks our cells. The immune system plays an important role in the body by fighting infections and allowing us to recover from illness. However, when an immune response is prolonged, it harms the body by attacking healthy cells like invading pathogens.

Suppose the parasympathetic nervous system does not effectively inhibit the immune system. In that case, chronic inflammation can lead to disorders in the tissues and organs and ultimately affect the physical and mental health of the person.

Autoimmune diseases

Autoimmune diseases occur when the immune system does not work properly but becomes overactive. In times of overactivity and runaway, the immune system attacks the body instead of toxins or dangerous substances. This directly damages the body, causing injury, inflammation, and pain.

This means that the best way to treat autoimmune disease is to slow down and reduce the immune system so that the flare-up of the autoimmune disease subsides and relief occurs. Some autoimmune diseases only cause problems in one area of the body, while others can affect all areas and cause discomfort and suffering. Regardless of the damage caused by the autoimmune disease you are suffering from, it is important to treat it to ensure that the body is maintained in the best possible condition.

Some of these tendencies to develop autoimmune diseases can be directly linked to genetics, with studies linking them to families. At the same time, diet and exercise are also thought to trigger autoimmune diseases. A final consideration as to why these diseases develop is what is known as the hygiene hypothesis. This hypothesis states that the immune system tends to overreact because children today are exposed to far fewer germs than in the past, because vaccinations have become commonplace, and because cleaning agents have been developed that kill the germs that children would otherwise have come into contact with. Since the immune system is no longer regularly stimulated, it becomes defective. Despite this theory, it is currently unknown what makes people susceptible to disorders or why they develop them. Chronic stress, our lifestyle, and unhealthy diet contribute to autoimmune diseases. It is one of the fastest-growing diseases in the United States. Examples of autoimmune diseases include rheumatoid arthritis, alopecia areata, Graves' disease, Hashimoto's thyroiditis, psoriasis, multiple sclerosis, Crohn's disease, systemic lupus erythematosus, type 1 diabetes, celiac disease, and many others.

Most of these health disorders start in the digestive tract, which is fitting because the digestive tract contains the largest population of immune cells. These cells are found here in large numbers because this is also the doorway for many toxins, pathogens, and chemicals into the body. The other entry point is the injured skin, which is less absorbent than the mouth and the digestive tract.

The immune cells are lined on the walls of the digestive tract. They are held in lymphatic tissue, constructed like pocket spaces, and called GALT.

The immune cells of the digestive tract encounter numerous invaders that they are supposed to fight. Constant exposure to these invading toxins and pathogens can desensitize the immune cells to them. Over a long period of time, they no longer react to the pathogens or fight them. They have worked so hard that they can no longer distinguish between the invaders and the immune cells. This is how autoimmune problems occur.

Some autoimmune diseases are hereditary but still need to be triggered first. As Hartmut Wekerle found in a 2016 review published in the journal Rheumatology, the following three factors contribute to the risk of developing an autoimmune disease:

- A lot of autoimmune, autoreactive T cells in the GALT
- An imbalance in the gut microbiome that promotes inflammation
- Hereditary genes that are prone to autoimmune diseases

We cannot do much against the first and the last factor. We don't know the number of autoimmune cells in the GALT, and we can't change our genes. What we can do is influence the second factor, which is the balance of the microbiome in the gut. We can do that by feeding the microbiome with the right foods.

Autoimmune diseases and the nervous system

Unfortunately, part of our work is geared toward what is best for our nervous system. We do absurd things like skipping dinner, gobbling down food, and running out the door without thinking about how it affects everything from memory to vitality. According to Dr. Porges, increasing autoimmunity and other natural disorders like fibromyalgia and dysautonomia are best classified as "the nervous system in a state of the barrier."

Avoiding endless stressors can improve our overall well-being by preventing our nervous system from becoming overwhelmed. The close relationship between the nervous system and the gut suggests that amplifying "invisible discomfort" is associated with the vagus nerve and the body's capacity (or lack thereof) to cope with stimuli that can naturally shut us down. The power of the polyvagal theory lies in its capacity to reveal a framework that enables us to gain a deeper understanding of how to manage and approach our nervous system within the context of human science that is not optimally equipped to handle the significant demands we impose on ourselves.

The vagus nerve and autoimmune diseases

Autoimmune diseases and the vagus nerve are linked in the same way as inflammation and the vagus nerve. This is partly because inflammation and autoimmune disease are inseparable - inflammation is an autoimmune response. You've heard of arthritis and diabetes, so you're familiar with autoimmune diseases. However, people can also suffer from a variety of other autoimmune diseases.
Immune disorders can be caused by an overactive immune system or a lack of immune system activity. In both cases, there are problems with the body's ability to manage its diseases because the defense systems fail in one way or another. As a result, part of the body fails to effectively fight the disease, infection, or another trigger for the body. There are over 80 different autoimmune diseases. Some are more common, while others are virtually unknown. 14 of the 80 are relatively common. However, in most cases, these diseases are common enough to mention, and people have at least heard of them. These 14 diseases include:

Rheumatoid arthritis: A disease in which the immune system attacks the joints, causing stiffness, pain, and inflammation in the affected joints.

Coeliac disease is when the immune system directly attacks the digestive system, leading to gastrointestinal sensitivity and inflammation.

Sjögren's syndrome: A disease in which the immune system attacks the glands in the eyes that produce the tear fluid. Dry eyes and a dry mouth most often manifest it.

Addison's disease: A disease in which the adrenal glands cannot produce the right number of hormones, leading to dysfunction in the body.

Hashimoto's thyroiditis: A disease in which the thyroid gland does not produce enough hormones. This leads to weight gain, intolerance to cold, swelling, and hair loss.

Psoriatic arthritis: A disease in which the immune system causes the skin to grow too fast - excess skin develops into inflamed and scaly patches. Arthritis sometimes accompanies this psoriasis and leads to joint pain and problems.

Pernicious anemia: A disease in which the body does not get enough protein and has difficulty making DNA effectively.

Inflammatory bowel disease: A disease commonly referred to as IBD, in which the immune system attacks the intestinal wall. This can occur in various forms, leading to inflammation of the gastrointestinal tract, resulting in pain and difficulty digesting food.

Autoimmune vasculitis: A disease in which the immune system attacks the blood vessels in the body, leading to inflammation of the vessels, causing the veins and arteries to narrow while making it difficult for blood to flow.

Multiple sclerosis: A disease in which the immune system attacks the brain - particularly the myelin sheath, the part of the neurons that sheathes the axon to help transmit the impulse. When this is damaged, the person's effectiveness in relaying messages decreases.

Graves' disease is when the immune system attacks the thyroid gland, causing too many hormones to be produced and released into the body. This can lead to high heart rates, difficulty tolerating heat, and unexplained weight loss.

Myasthenia Gravis: A disease in which the immune system damages the way the brain communicates with the muscles by affecting the nerves that transmit from the mind to the body, resulting in muscle weakening that seems to worsen the more actions are taken performed.

Systemic lupus erythematosus: A disease in which the immune system attacks a large part of the body, affecting the brain, joints, various organs, and even the heart. It causes skin rashes, pain, and fatigue.

Type 1 diabetes: A disease in which the immune system attacks cells in the pancreas responsible for producing insulin so that the body can no longer process glucose effectively.

However, stimulation of the vagus nerve has been shown to help inhibit inflammation, which in turn should help alleviate some of the autoimmune response. When inflammation is contained, the body no longer sends signals to fight parts of the body where immune system intervention is unnecessary.

The afferent pathway, the pathway from the body to the brain, tells the body if an injury or if an immune response is necessary. It has been shown that the body can regulate itself when the afferent nerve is blocked in some way, but the efferent pathway can continue normally or is even stimulated. Communication between the brain and the body continues. In contrast, the brain is prevented from producing more pro-inflammatory hormones because it is not receiving the impulses that tell the brain that inflammation is occurring. By blocking the afferent impulses and promoting them, the body can regulate itself - it stops producing the cytokines that cause further inflammation, which is responsible for the immune system attacking the body.

Living with an autoimmune disease

The first signs of an autoimmune disease may be general, such as exhaustion, fever, and difficulty concentrating, which makes it difficult to diagnose autoimmune diseases from the start. You may also feel discouraged and seek help from an expert.

Overproduction of cytokines and chemokines leads to inflammation of the body tissue in autoimmune diseases. A high concentration of cytokines in the joints can cause rheumatoid arthritis, for example. This condition worsens when chemokines attract other harmful immune system components, such as macrophages, neutrophils, and T-cells, into the joint, exacerbating the inflammatory response.

Multiple sclerosis, the best-known nerve disease in young adults, is a permanent disorder of the nervous system believed to be caused by a confusing autoimmune attack on myelin, a protective covering of nerve cells. In multiple sclerosis, the myelin is gradually dissolved by the body's immune system, leading to difficulties with muscle coordination (because muscles require nerve activity) and vision. As the disease progresses, the inflammation decreases for unknown reasons, but the body tissue is damaged in the long term. Experts believe that the autoimmune trigger in multiple sclerosis is a disease caused by an infection or other microorganisms, but this has not been proven.

Nourishing our bodies is crucial for recovery and rebuilding vagal tone. In our go-go-go culture of momentary gratification and glorification of the takeaway, ensuring that body and psyche are in sync is essential for wellbeing. Currently, it is more palpable than ever that the cure for actually existing around lived untruths is to find a balance between the many interrelated needs of life and to become aware of one's own body and the physiological state changes that affect oneself (and others!) much more than we commonly think.

Chapter 5: Symptoms of Vagus Nerve Dysfunction

Due to the role of the vagus nerve in the parasympathetic nervous system and its effect on vital organs of the body, such as the heart, lungs, and intestines, this nerve is of great importance for our general health and well-being.

Any disturbance of the vagus nerve can have far-reaching consequences for the entire body and lead to a plethora of diseases and health problems. It is essential to understand that most of the conditions discussed here do not exist separately, meaning that if one of these diseases is present in the human body, it can lead to other diseases. For example, obesity and inflammation are associated with cancer and diabetes, and anxiety and mood disorders can also lead to depression.

Some of the signs that can be associated with poor vagus nerve function are:

Trauma, Depression, and PTSD

Witnessing a traumatic experience such as a natural disaster, an act of violence, abuse, or even a severe accident can have an impact on mental health and lead to mental disorders. We will have some degree of emotional reaction whether we are directly affected by such experiences, have family members or friends who have been affected (killed or injured), or learn about the event through the media. Regardless of the nature of the trauma, it can have long-term psychological effects on a person.

Our feelings due to traumatic events (such as sadness, mood swings, crying, social withdrawal, etc.) are part of the normal grieving and recovery process. However, suppose these feelings continue unchecked for a long time and start interfering with your daily life. In that case, if you begin to use alcohol or illegal drugs or even think about suicide, these are symptoms of more severe depression.

Dysfunctional breathing

Most of us unconsciously take our breathing for granted because we know "how we breathe" rather than "how we should breathe." Unfortunately, dysfunctional breathing is one of the most common causes of vagus nerve dysfunction. Breathing correctly is one of the most effortless things you can do for your health, yet many find it difficult. In the following sections, where I focus on strengthening vagal tone, I will describe how you can learn to breathe correctly to live a better and healthier life.

Lack of social interaction

Face-to-face social contact stimulates the vagus nerve and increases the parasympathetic nervous system, positively affecting health. Imagine being cut off from others for a week or more or staying indoors without contact with the outside world, your family members, partners, or even close friends; you would most likely become depressed and moody. This is not a random sensation; the vagus nerve is activated when interacting with people face to face and deactivated when you are alone. In addition, social contact improves heart rate variability (HRV), which indicates a high vagal tone.

Chronic nausea

When your body cannot digest your food properly, it may resort to making do with what it has. Consequently, if your body detects that you consistently consume more food than is necessary, you may experience symptoms such as nausea triggered by the mere thought or scent of food. These symptoms manifest your body's effort to prevent you from overburdening it.

Weight loss

In stressful situations, the weight loss is quite dramatic, and it is almost exclusively the muscle mass that is lost. Unfortunately, this drastically reduces strength, which only causes the body to store more fat. The result is a "skinny-fat" look, where a person looks weak all around but has large amounts of fat stored in the middle, causing the belly to stand out unmistakably.

Dysfunctional digestive system

When the vagus nerve is disturbed, your digestive system is at risk of malfunctioning. For example, Heartburn or gastroesophageal reflux disease (GERD) and inflammatory bowel disease (IBD) such as ulcerative colitis, which can prevent the body from healing small intestinal bacterial overgrowth (SIBO), a common cause of IBS, are some symptoms of the impaired digestive system (IBS).

The vagus nerve instructs your stomach to release digestive acids and enzymes and initiate the digestive process. For example, when you chew your food, you combine the fibers with the digestive acids and enzymes that break down the food before it reaches your stomach and enters your small and large intestines.

If the vagus nerve does not receive or transmit the right signals, the flow of food, digestive acid, and enzymes through the intestine is throttled. As a result, bacteria, yeast, parasites, and spent hormones and toxins that the body has diligently removed from the system move slowly through the gut. Exposing your body to these bacteria increases the likelihood of developing IBS and SIBO, which can most likely aggravate infections already in your body.

Weight gain

All the fat that the person accumulates will eventually show up on the scale. The person may regain their original weight after losing weight, but their body shape will change emphatically. They have inherited the worst of all worlds because a lot of muscle has been lost and replaced by fat. They no longer have the strength to perform tasks that they used to be able to do with their eyes closed, and they are now even heavier, which adds to their problems.

Cardiovascular problems

An increase in weight and a decrease in strength indicate that the heart is functioning with reduced efficiency in terms of circulating blood throughout the body. This is compounded by the additional strain of supplying a larger mass, resulting in one of two potential issues. Either the heart begins to beat excessively fast, known as tachycardia, or it slows down significantly, referred to as bradycardia.

Heartburn

This is because your gut microbiome is decimated, so your body cannot digest many foods. The result is heartburn and hyperacidity. Hypersensitivity to acid reflux is called heartburn. We all have experienced that burning sensation in the throat after eating certain foods. This burning sensation is typically our body's reaction to excessive acid in the digestive tract.

The vagus nerve plays a central role in communication between the gut and the brain. When this communication pathway is disrupted, the regulation of the gut can be impaired, leading to an accumulation of acid and, subsequently, heartburn.

Dizziness

If your heart health deteriorates, your blood pressure will vary more. As a result, you will feel weak if you change your position suddenly, for example, if you stand up immediately after sitting for a while.

Sleep disorders and disturbance of the circadian rhythm

A common problem I have observed in people is a disruption in their body's natural sleep signaling or circadian rhythm. This is partly because most people are no longer physically active during the day. We only see the sun occasionally during the day. When we get home at night, we sit directly in front of blue lights on our mobile phones, computers, or even our televisions, which falsely fool our brains into thinking it's daytime. The blue light emitted from the screens of our electronic devices mimics the sun, tells our bodies it's time to wake up, and instructs the pineal glands in our brains not to release melatonin (a sleep-inducing hormone).

The vagus nerve transmits signals from our circadian control center, located high up in our brain. Disruption of circadian flow affects the brain, and changes in melatonin levels and other hormones just before bedtime can cause difficulties with the vagus nerve.

Dysfunctional heart rate

The number of heartbeats per minute is called heart rate and is directly related to the heart's workload during daily activities.
When the body is at rest (i.e., relaxed for a period of time), the resting heart rate can be measured. The average resting heart rate for most people is in the range of 60-100 beats per minute (bpm). However, in athletes, it is customary to be between 40 and 60 beats per minute. A dysfunctional heart rate or abnormal heart rhythm describes a heart that beats too fast (over 100 beats per minute) or too slow (under 60 beats per minute).

Chronic fatigue

Fatigue is a physical and mental debilitation characterized by a general lack of motivation and energy. While it is normal to feel tired after a long day of work or intense physical activity, chronic fatigue is characterized by a lack of energy and a general malaise that cannot be traced to a single source.
If you suffer from chronic fatigue, you will find that you are tired as soon as you wake up in the morning. You feel listless throughout the day and may even feel like you don't want to do anything. If you are constantly tired, have little energy, and don't feel like going about your day, even if you have just woken up, you should have the well-being of your vagus nerve checked. An infection of the vagus nerve can lead to chronic fatigue.

Irritable bowel syndrome

The vagus nerve plays an essential role in enabling digestive functions, and when it is not working properly, abdominal disorders can become a possible symptom. In addition, infection of the cells lining the digestive tract can lead to intestinal irritation due to persistent fight-or-flight response activation.
When the vagus nerve does its job correctly, it has an anti-inflammatory effect by inhibiting sympathetic responses. However, when the vagus nerve is not functioning properly, the sympathetic responses are prolonged, leading to inflammation.

Chronic stress and anxiety

In life, there are ups and downs. Many experiences and situations trigger anxiety in the average person, from work-related stress to relationship problems and family dysfunction. In most cases, you should be able to deal with anxiety as it comes and goes. However, if you are constantly fearful, this could indicate that your vagus nerve is not functioning correctly.

The function of the vagus nerve is to put the body in a relaxed state and promote self-soothing, which ensures that we are not constantly agitated. Stress triggers our sympathetic nervous system, which prepares us for flight or fight by stimulating our body to act. To bring the body back to a relaxed state after arousal, the parasympathetic responses of the vagus nerve must override the reactions of the sympathetic nervous system.

This means that the vagus nerve should be able to slow down your heartbeat and breathing rate so that you feel calm and liberated. If the parasympathetic mechanism of the vagus nerve is not working correctly, you are prone to chronic anxiety, which can lead to chronic inflammation or even depression.

Chronic inflammations

Chronic inflammation is usually a clue that our immune system is overstimulated. As a result of its persistent action, the body begins to fight its cells, leading to chronic inflammation. When your vagus nerve is functioning correctly, it can turn off the persistent response of the immune system by preventing the release of tumor necrosis factor and causing the release of acetylcholine. When set in motion by the vagus nerve, these two mechanisms effectively inhibit inflammation. However, this is only possible if the vagus nerve is functioning properly.

Chronic inflammation can cause severe physical and mental distress, and increasingly vagus nerve therapy is being used to alleviate the effects of inflammation in conditions such as rheumatoid arthritis and epilepsy.

Chapter 6: How to stimulate the vagus nerve?

There are a lot of possibilities for activating the vagus nerve. You can choose the ones that pique your interest. The important thing is that you like what you have chosen so that you can stick with it and ensure that you are beneficially practicing vagus stimulation.

These methods will teach you to interact with your body. For example, you could go for a walk to activate the vagus nerve. Others prefer methods that do not require a device implanted in the body, such as massaging the vagus nerve or some other type of stimulation.

These methods are great for transforming your mind quickly and easily if you already have a way to influence it directly. For example, you could practice yoga at home to stretch the vagus nerve and activate it that way. However, whatever method you use, it should have the desired effect. This is because your mind changes when your body changes.

Regarding the methods you can use, the possibilities are almost unlimited. Anything that directly changes one thing or another by activating the vagus nerve can be considered. Some of the most common methods are:

Meditation

Meditation is an extremely powerful state of mind and has been found to stimulate the same brain regions as the vagus nerve, suggesting that the two are connected.

When you meditate, you enter a calm, stable state where you can relax and focus on your feelings. You focus on the clarity and peace within yourself and can thus gradually but steadily find comfort within yourself.

Sometimes people resist meditation, but the truth is that it is remarkably effective. You don't have to give up everything you enjoy to meditate. On the contrary, you can usually do it anywhere and for any length of time with minimal effort. All you need is yourself and a quiet place where you can pause, undisturbed and alone, to find inner peace.

First, find a nice, quiet place to relax without being disturbed. Then, ensure it is a place where you can concentrate better without distractions.

Breathe in deeply and hold your breath. Then breathe out. Repeat this step and get used to how your breath feels.

Find a posture that you like to sit in. It can be any position; it doesn't have to be any particular one. The important thing is that you feel comfortable in it.

Slowly focus your attention on your breathing. At this point, focus only on your breathing and pay attention to the air flowing in and out of your lungs.

Each time you feel your attention leaving your breathing, you must bring it back quietly and gently, free from judgment and worry.

Stay in this phase for as long as you feel comfortable, preferably at least five minutes.

How you meditate is up to you, but many people enjoy listening to soft music while letting their minds wander and focusing on their breath.

Emptying your mind can be a clearing experience and can make you feel calmer and more centered as you go about your day. If you suffer from anxiety and stress, meditation can help reduce the impact on your body and calm you down before you get on with what you need to get done. It also lets you focus on the task rather than what happened earlier.

If you find meditation unclear or complex, take a guided meditation that you can listen to while you perfect your technique. There are several free ones on YouTube that you can take advantage of. Meditation has the added benefit of using chanting or breathing techniques to help you relax. At the same time, you are using another excellent method to activate your vagus nerve. You will also have more drive and feel more balanced after a meditation session.

Cold exposure

You may have heard cold showers or baths are good for you, but did you know cold activates your vagus nerve? It also affects the cholinergic neurons along the vagus nerve. Cold exposure stimulates the nerve and helps to tighten it, making it more efficient.

You can reduce stress or anxiety by decreasing the sympathetic nervous system's response to stressors. Exposure to cold can increase parasympathetic nervous system activity, which helps limit the fight-or-flight response. It can also help to reduce stomach problems. If you are feeling ill, spending time in the cold can often reverse the feeling of nausea.

There are various methods of cold exposure. There's the infamous plunge into an icy lake, but something easier is to take a cold shower or even pour cold water on your face. You might start slowly, setting the shower to cold for just the last minute, and gradually work your way up to a completely cold shower. However you do it, you will notice the improvements in your health in a few weeks.

Some people enjoy going outside in winter without wrapping up, and this can be a great way to expose yourself to the cold. Just a few minutes can affect the vagus nerve and improve your situation.

Studies have shown that cold is most effective on the back of the neck. So try putting a cold flannel on the back of your neck for the best results.

Any acute exposure to cold leads to increased stimulation of the vagus nerve. Scientific studies show that the body's tendency to flee or fight (sympathetic nervous system) decreases, and the tendency to rest and digest (parasympathetic nervous system) increases when the body is exposed to cold, the latter mediated by the vagus nerve. This includes immersing the face in cold water, drinking cold liquids, or using a cold waistcoat. Cold showers are also very accessible and extremely useful. Cold water has many benefits and advantages for the human body. Cold water therapies are known to prolong the response to shock and stressful situations and can simultaneously trigger flight and fight hormones. These triggers are particularly beneficial when you are faced with danger or have to deal with some stress. You need to prepare your response system for them to ensure that these events do not bring you down or put you in a heart failure state.

The effects of cold water on the vagus nerve also go so far as to affect the immune system. Studies have been conducted to varying degrees to investigate the relationship between cold water and the immune system. These studies have shown that the immune system can be strengthened when the body is exposed to cold water. The experiment was conducted with some people who had volunteered. They wanted to know how to control their nervous reactions.

It is a well-known fact that the body's involuntary reactions cannot be controlled. Some of these involuntary reactions are breathing, heartbeat, the release of hormones, and many more. However, we have seen that people who spend time in meditation and yoga classes have already achieved this control. They have learned over time how to bring the body into total control, where every response to a stimulus is self-determined. Science has been somewhat reticent about this theory but later gained concrete insights into how these actions are possible.

Humming and singing

When you hum or sing, the air passes through the folds of your lips and causes a vibration. This vibration is what creates the audible sounds in your mouth. As a form of stress relief therapy, doctors advise singing and making melodies when you feel you are starting to get depressed, anxious, or stressed. This works because the vagus folds, which vibrate along with the muscles, also cause the vagus nerve to vibrate. This vibration helps the nerve to receive the signal and transmit it as it should. Imagine a metal whose vibration rubs off on another metal nearby, causing both to vibrate to each other. Humming and singing have also been shown to help stabilize the heart rate and improve the vagal tone.

Uplifting singing, mantra chanting, humming, and hymn singing all increase heart rate variability (HRV) in different ways. Singing from the top of the lungs challenges the muscles in the back of the throat, activating the vagus nerve. So the next time you are caught singing along to the radio while driving, tell him you are only exercising and stimulating the vagus nerve.

Singing is like activating a vagus pump that sends out waves of relaxation. Whether you sing alone or together (in a church or with a group of friends) doesn't matter. In both cases, the function of the vagus nerve is activated, relaxation is increased, the mood is lifted, and heart rate variability (HRV) is also increased.

Gargle

The technique of gargling was made famous by Dr. Datis Kharrazian. It simply involves pouring a liquid (e.g., water) into the mouth and the back of the throat while aggressively moving it to make a gurgling sound.

When you gargle, the pharyngeal muscles (the muscles at the back of the throat) contract, activating the vagus nerve - often called a "sprint" for the vagus nerve. For gargling to be effective, you need to gargle aggressively and loudly until tears come to your eyes, and if they don't, keep doing it until they do. This indicates that you have activated your vagus nerve. This can be difficult initially, especially if your vagal tone is low. The idea is to gargle for up to 5 minutes thrice daily. Then, start with a shorter time and gradually increase it. Adding salt to the water before gargling has been shown to have an antibacterial effect that can help eliminate unwanted bacteria from the mouth and respiratory tract. Gargling daily can help increase the responsiveness of the vagus nerve, which regulates relaxation, metabolism, and digestion. It has also been shown to improve memory.

Gargling is an excellent way to stimulate the vagus nerve. Why is this the case? First, it helps to vibrate the vocal folds and muscles, which affects the vagal nerve.

When you want to gargle, put some water in your mouth (a small amount you can swallow without spilling). Make sure your head is tilted upwards so the water stays in your mouth while you open it. This way, you make the water vibrate in your mouth by vibrating your vocal muscles. It looks more like you are trying to make sounds while the water is still in your mouth. If you do it right, you should make a childlike sound, similar to how children brush their teeth. Doing this repeatedly for a few minutes will stimulate your vagus nerve.

You can also do this exercise as a form of release. Just the thought that you are doing this exercise is liberating. While you gargle with the water in your mouth, you switch off all the fantasies running through your head. You will feel more relief than you expected. As your vocal folds begin to vibrate, they send waves down the vagus nerve and back into the throat. This constant activity wakes up all the dormant areas of the nerve. Because the nerve is made up of a long connection of neurons, certain regions of the nerve endings may have become numb and cold. The waves sent by the vibration help to restore each part of the connection.

Laughter

Laughter is a straightforward way to stimulate the vagus nerve. It is a natural immune stimulator for the body, which research shows also increases heart rate variability (HRV). Laughter boosts the movement of the diaphragm and pressure on the abdomen (stomach). Since the vagus nerve runs from the brain stem through the diaphragm, these movements activate the parasympathetic nervous system, which sends signals to the body to relax. When you laugh, you usually crank up your rest, digestive, and nervous systems to reduce your stress hormones and release your body's painkillers, such as endorphins (a feel-good hormone). Laughter has also been shown to be beneficial for cognitive function and protects against heart disease. It improves beta-endorphins and nitric oxide levels and positively affects the vascular system. It has also been shown that those who enact funny scenarios generally have lower cortisol levels.

Start by laughing at something funny. For example, watch an online comedy show, read a comic book, or take turns telling jokes to a friend or a child. You will soon find yourself laughing and experiencing an improved mood and vagal tone.

Resolve to laugh daily to give yourself an inner massage and stimulate the vagus nerve. We should all be able to laugh at least a few times a day heartily. If you don't, it's time to change something in your life. A reliable way to start is by attending a comedy show, watching a comedy film, or simply sharing jokes with family and friends. You don't have to laugh out loud to experience the beneficial effects of laughter when your vagus nerve is stimulated. You can also find something in your office that makes you laugh, such as watching a funny TV program, reading a comic book, or doing anything that makes you laugh inside - all of which are just as therapeutic as laughing out loud.

Fasting

Intermittent fasting helps you to increase higher frequency pulse rate variability, which is a marker of vagal tone. When you fast, part of the decrease in metabolic rate is mediated by the vagus nerve as it detects a reduction in blood glucose levels along with a decrease in chemical and mechanical stimuli from the gut (reference).

Food in a quiet state

Do not eat breakfast in a hurry or eat lunch at work or dinner in front of the computer. Eating a meal in a hectic environment can have harmful and long-lasting consequences. Eating in a peaceful environment and a state of personal calm is important. Choose a delicious meal, chew the food properly, and relax.

The basic act of chewing food causes the stomach to secrete acid, bile formation in the liver, and the release of bile in the gallbladder to be triggered, stomach enzymes to be secreted from the pancreas, and intestinal motility to be transmitted through the vagus nerve.

Therefore, it is important to put digestion in the right order, and the body will do this automatically if you start the procedure correctly. Before swallowing, you should have time to chew the food until it is mushy and soft. This sets the correct sequence of digestion in motion and allows the vagus nerve to perform its activities properly. If you stick to these habits and exercises, you will feel better and see the world in a relaxed, calm, and pleasant state.

Breathing to stimulate the vagus nerve

Have you ever noticed that your breathing speeds up when you are scared? This is because of your sympathetic nervous system - your body goes into a fight-flight-freeze mode to survive. So when you want to calm down after a panic attack, you may instinctively do deep breathing exercises to regulate yourself. Do you understand why? Most people don't know that deep breathing signals to the vagus nerve that it's time to get to work. As the vagus nerve activates the parasympathetic nervous system, it is essentially triggered to act in a way that can alleviate symptoms and slow the heart rate.

The vagus nerve is stimulated by deep and slow breathing. In the neck and center of the body, baroreceptors or stretch receptors detect blood pressure and send the necessary signals to the brain. These signals activate the vagus nerve, causing blood pressure and pulse rate to drop. As a result, the sympathetic fight and flight response is reduced, and the parasympathetic sleep and digestive response are increased. Slower breathing increases awareness of these receptors, resulting in increased vagal activation. An important note: Breathe gradually and allow your abdomen to rise and fall. This is a conscious diaphragmatic muscle action. Your traps and shoulders should not move much with each breath as secondary respiratory muscles control these actions. The deeper you breathe, the more your abdomen expands and contracts. Have you ever noticed how your heartbeat changes when you breathe? When you take a deep breath, you may feel your pulse quicken, and when you exhale, you notice it slow down again. A particular reason for this is that your vagus nerve regulates your heart rate. When you inhale, your pulse speeds up, and when your pulse speeds up, your blood pressure increases.

This increase in blood pressure and pulse triggers the parasympathetic nervous system - it wants to regulate the heart rate, releasing some acetylcholine into the bloodstream and throttling the heart rate. It means that you can effectively engage your vagus nerve by simply taking a deep breath and signaling to the nerve that you need to regulate your heart rate. When you exhale, your vagus nerve is most active and effectively slows your heart rate. This means you can effectively regulate yourself and your parasympathetic nervous system through breathing.

This is nothing new because the breathing pattern that triggers this calm state, thanks to the parasympathetic nervous system, occurs during various calming, spiritual activities. Mantras can trigger this activation in any meditation by establishing and maintaining the right timing between breaths, as can praying the Hail Mary. The breathing rate is lowered to about six breaths per minute, which is the aim of these breathing techniques.

Socialization to stimulate the vagus nerve

The ability to socialize is increased by activity in the ventral system. The good news is that this connection works both ways. When you set out to socialize, your brain recognizes it is not dangerous and automatically activates the ventral system.

The term "relationship" might confuse you here. The term I use here applies to romantic and platonic relationships. It even covers situations that do not fall into either category. For example, something as simple as small talk with a stranger can make your brain realize that the situation is not full of danger.

Therefore, depression forces you to isolate yourself because it is simply a reaction to how the nervous system perceives the environment. It is preoccupied with survival and therefore does not value social connections. Bringing this to the forefront forces your brain to re-evaluate the situation. It would help to use this very powerful technique as often as possible.

We return to the social nervous system, the proposed technique by which the vagus nerve regulates how we socialize. It has been shown that social contact is one of the best ways to relieve stress, and that makes sense. Think about it - we are social creatures. You need to be with people you love and care about to relieve stress. Moreover, this socializing can make you feel fulfilled and better than ever.

Many of you say that the only way to get your anxiety or depression back under control is to make sure you go out. You have to reboot the mind, so to speak, so that it finds it beneficial and advantageous - does that sound familiar?

Even if you only spend a few minutes every day talking to someone in the café while you wait for your order, you will come into contact with other people, and when they talk to you, you will find that you can gradually function again. You will be able to feel comfortable in your own body again.

When interacting with another person, there are many ways to increase the benefits of vagal tone for both of you. First, build a meaningful, connected relationship with the other person. This will help you both. Eye contact and physical closeness can also be helpful. Hugs are an excellent way to stimulate the vagus nerve through physical pressure and positive associations.

You have probably noticed that it just feels good when someone hugs you. Of course, some people are better at hugging than others. Still, the connection is strengthened by hugs and physical contact, which makes it more possible for you to continue the relationship and see it in a positive light. All this is good for vagal tone and should be maintained if possible.

Relaxing to stimulate the vagus nerve

When you are relaxed, your vagus nerve is naturally stimulated. It is responsible for the feeling of relaxation when nothing else is going on. You feel this when you curl up in bed or on the sofa with a cozy blanket and your favorite book. The vagus nerve is effectively stimulated even when you can relax without worrying about anything. If you do this regularly, you know you can strengthen your vagus nerve.

Remember that this is a lifestyle change. The vagus nerve will only stay as tight as you can hold it if you continue to stimulate it after the point. As with any other body part, the same applies here: If you don't use it, you will lose it. So you must remember to maintain your lifestyle as long as you expect your vagus tone to improve.

Remember that it's up to you at the end of the day. It is up to you to better manage the stress in your life, and if you want the added benefit of turning it off, then you must be willing to make an effort.

Exercise

Health experts have found that exercise stimulates the vagus nerve by increasing the heart rate, thus improving parasympathetic activity and training the body to recover easily from exertion.

Apart from the numerous effects exercise has on the health of the body, the contribution it makes to the development of a healthy brain and mind is a benefit we cannot overlook. For this reason, you should make an effort to exercise regularly, at least once a day. If your daily routine does not allow this, you can limit yourself to 4 times a week. When you exercise, your sweat pores open up so that waste products can be released as sweat. If you do this regularly, you will notice an increase in the nervous system in your body. Sticking to routine exercises that make you feel comfortable is more advisable.

Any kind of exercise can be beneficial, so pick something you enjoy. If you like the movement, you will be more likely to keep it up. Some activities you may want to try are:

- Go for a walk: Walking through the park or around the block can significantly increase your activity level.
- Swimming: This is a gentle exercise for people with limited mobility that strengthens the muscles.
- Cycling: Get on a bike and pedal to increase your lung capacity, lose weight and strengthen your nervous system.
- Hiking: This is also an excellent way to socialize because hiking is best done with friends.
- Running/jogging: You don't necessarily have to run a marathon (although that's fun), but moving fast will increase your vagal tone.
- Weightlifting: If you don't enjoy exercising, try weightlifting to strengthen both the muscles and the vagus nerve.
- Yoga: Strengthen your body with stretching exercises and add some social elements when attending a class.
- Aerobics: Another good way to exercise is to take an aerobics class or video class at home.
- Dancing: Who doesn't love to dance? Go to the clubs or stay home and dance around the house.
- Kayaking: Get out on the water and move around to increase vagal tone.
- Martial arts: You can learn to defend yourself and increase your vagus tone at the same time.
- Gymnastics: You learn to stretch and move, so it's a two-for-one deal.
- Team sports: If you enjoy playing basketball, football, or anything else, you'll find that playing a sport in a team gives you a natural energy boost.

There are no limits to the types of exercise you can try. If something doesn't work for you, change sports.

If you find it hard to exercise, even if it is something you enjoy, you can keep it up in a few ways. First, there is nothing wrong with a little extra motivation to keep you moving.

Find a training partner to support you. It is constructive to exercise with someone, even if it is just a walking partner. If you make an appointment to work with someone, you are more likely to keep the agreement so you don't bail out at the last minute. Alternatively, have someone you check in with every day, even if they are far away. In this way, if you have to report, you have a better reason to keep your commitments.

Sign up for courses. If you spend money on classes, you will probably attend them. After all, you don't want to waste money. Just make sure it is something you really want to do. For example, there is little point in taking a karate course if you hate martial arts. There are so many different sports courses that there is always something to learn.

Join a team. Do you really need some motivation? Join a sports team. Whether you want to play baseball or go dragon boating, a team will keep you going when you don't want to move because other people depend on you. A team sport can be fun for competitive people and might even get you moving more than usual.

Hire a trainer. A personal trainer comes at an extra cost, but if you can afford it, you'll have someone to push you to your physical limits. I have found that a personal trainer has actually helped me to overcome the training gap. When I couldn't push myself, having someone push me was helpful.

Get a dog. A dog is not only a great companion and gives unconditional love, but it also needs to be walked. You can't skip walks as this can lead to chaos in the house. However, the extra motivation to get out could be just what you need to get moving.

Rewarding yourself when you achieve a set goal, such as running a certain distance at a particular time or lifting a certain weight, can also be helpful. You can choose the reward yourself, but it should keep you motivated.

The saliva exercise stimulates the vagus nerve

If you currently have post-traumatic stress disorder, you can calm yourself down again with the help of saliva. I know it may seem strange, but you can free yourself from shock or anxiety by forcing yourself to salivate. Regardless of whether you are in a state of fight, flight, or freeze, activating the vagus nerve through salivation reminds your mind that all is well.

You can stop and remind yourself that you will be fine if you pay attention to what is happening around you and start to trigger your behaviors. Since the body does not naturally salivate when stressed or under attack, you can remind your body that there are no current threats in your immediate environment by making yourself salivate. You can remind yourself that there is no reason to be afraid; basically, you remind yourself to calm down and avoid worrying too much about what is happening.

It's very easy to do. Just follow the steps below:

Take a deep breath and close your eyes.

- Let your tongue relax in your mouth, the tip pressed against the inside of the lowest teeth.
- Imagine that you are holding your favorite food in your hand. It can be anything; imagine that you are holding it in your hand and about to bite. Please pay attention to how it looks. Pay attention to how the texture looks. Imagine how it smells and how it will feel in your mouth when you finally bite into it.
- In response to the images in your head, you should start salivating. First, make sure that the saliva collects in your mouth. There should be a small puddle in the lower part of your mouth.
- Let your tongue bathe in the saliva for a few minutes with your eyes closed. After that, you should begin to feel calmer.

The diving reflex stimulates the vagus nerve

This is a natural human reflex that changes how the body functions immediately. It is typically triggered when one is fully immersed in water, especially cold water, and results in a sudden cessation of breathing, a slowing of the heartbeat, and an attempt to restrict blood flow from the limbs to the vital organs and brain.

This is essentially the body's attempt to shut down as much of itself as possible after water immersion to conserve vital resources. These are resources like the oxygen that the body needs.

But what does this reflex sound like? First, you see a cessation of breathing and a lightning-like reduction in heart rate thanks to the vagus nerve. This means that by triggering your diving reflex, you can activate your vagus nerve so that your body slows down. All you have to do to do this is:

- Open the tap in the sink and let the water run as cold as possible.
- Put the water in your hand and splash it on your face when it is cold. To trigger this effect properly, the water should hit everywhere, from the hairline to the lips. While splashing the water on your face, you should also hold your breath.
- Hold this for a moment and enjoy the benefits it brings.
- The diving reflex refers to how our body reacts when submerged in water. Our brain gets more blood flow, and our senses are heightened. You don't have to jump into the water to achieve this effect. Splash cold water on your face, and you will feel the effect.

Another way to create this effect is to hold a pack of ice cubes in front of your face and hold your breath for a few seconds. A third method is to drink water and play with it as it flows over your tongue and you feel its texture.

Taking care of a small child

Immediately after birth, mothers experience a surge of hormones, including oxytocin, which promotes bonding with their newborns. The same hormone is also released during positive social interactions. Parents benefit from a close relationship with their babies and children, but you can also enjoy these benefits without a child.
Researchers found that caring for children can stimulate and improve the tone of the vagus nerve. Caring for young children is a good start, and you will probably get lots of hugs and kisses. All this physical contact will undoubtedly positively affect your vagal tone. Babysitting is an excellent opportunity to gain experience in caring for children.

Babies and young children are great for your vagus nerve, but you can also benefit from caring for animals or some older people. Consider volunteering at a nursing home, as a caregiver, or in another position where you can help care for people or things. This will help you release more oxytocin, improve your vagal tone and do some good for the world at the same time.

Sex

We have a sex drive for a reason, and apart from reproductive purposes, sex can be an excellent way to stimulate the vagus nerve. Any activity that targets the pelvis can activate the vagus nerve, and sex is the ultimate way to target the pelvis and stimulate the various nerve endings there.

However, sex is not just about pleasure and orgasm; these are outstanding opportunities to increase vagal tone. In addition, when you have sexual intercourse or even foreplay with someone, you participate in social interaction and a very intimate way of connecting with another person. Therefore, this practice can double affect vagal tone and make you feel happier and calmer.

Of course, this doesn't mean you should have sex with everyone. Even masturbation techniques can give you half the equation and increase your vagal tone. However, if you have someone special to enjoy intimate hours with, you will definitely notice the benefits over time.

Coffee Enemas

When you think of stimulating the vagus nerve, enemas are probably not the first thing that comes to mind, but they can be very effective. After all, the vagus nerve is particularly influenced by the bowel, and when you use it, you also activate the vagus nerve.

A coffee enema is used to cleanse the bowels and relieve constipation. During a coffee enema, the caffeine stimulates the release of cholinergic receptors (especially the nicotinic receptor) in the bowel, which in turn promotes the movement and expansion of the bowel and activates the vagus nerve. This is particularly effective when consuming a high concentration of caffeine, which triggers a strong urge to urinate. The most important thing is to resist the urge and hold it in as long as possible. By resisting the urge, you train your brain and vagus nerve to learn to stimulate bowel motility. If you do this regularly with a coffee enema, your vagus nerve will eventually learn to release stool from the bowel without a coffee enema. This can be tedious initially, especially if your vagal tone is low, but it will become easier over time. If you suffer from chronic constipation and poor liver detoxification, taking a coffee enema and resisting the urge will undoubtedly help detoxify your body and empty your bowels very efficiently.

Enemas on the vagus nerve are similar to sprints. As with enemas, the vagus nerve is activated more effectively when the bowel is stretched. This happens by increasing the liver's ability to detoxify toxins in the blood and bind them to the bile. The liver cleanses itself by draining toxic bile into the small and large intestines. The entire bloodstream circulates through the liver every three minutes. Taking caffeine for 12 to 15 minutes allows the blood to flow through the liver four or five times, similar to dialysis treatment. The water content of coffee stimulates intestinal peristalsis and helps to expel toxic bile stored in the colon.

Coffee can be used to give yourself an enema that stimulates the vagus nerve. Any liquid will help, but coffee is the most effective because it contains compounds that stimulate nerve endings. It also stimulates the bile ducts, which aids digestion.

Enemas, including those with coffee, help flush toxins from the intestines. This reduces inflammation and helps improve vagal tone. You can make your enema from cool coffee or buy ready-made bottled enemas that are easy to use. If you make your own enema, stick to one teaspoon of coffee grounds per enema, as it can be too intense to use all the coffee.

Acupressure and acupuncture

Acupuncture and acupressure are very similar, except that one method uses pressure, and the other uses very thin needles to stimulate specific pressure points. Both techniques can be used to stimulate the vagus nerve and increase the parasympathetic response physically. Therefore, they are considered a recognized alternative to the enema described above.

Inserting needles or applying pressure to specific points in the body can stimulate the vagus nerve and quickly improve its tone. This procedure can be done in any practice, and the therapist should know exactly which points to use to stimulate the function of the nerve.

Each of these methods can be done easily and will not harm you. However, if you are serious about activating your vagus nerve, I recommend choosing three or four of these activities and scheduling them into your daily routine. It should not take too long, and the results can be extraordinary.

Standard acupuncture and ear acupuncture stimulate the activity of the vagus nerve. The positive effects of acupuncture are now widely recognized, partly because you can ask almost anyone who has had such a treatment and hear about its calming effect and the restful thoughts people have after an acupuncture treatment. I know that many of my patients are thrilled.

Electrical stimulation

This practice involves stimulating the vagus nerve by implanting a clinical device in the chest that sends electrical impulses to the brain. The FDA has approved this device to treat nervous system disorders such as seizures and depression.

This device is surgically implanted into the body just under the skin on the chest, where it is connected to the vagus nerve on the left side of the body. Electrical signals are sent to the brain via the vagus nerve when the device is switched on.

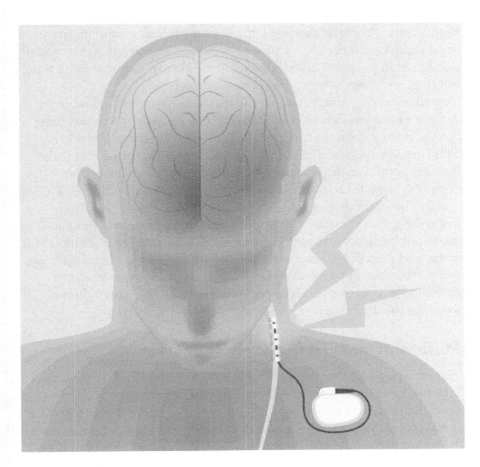

In recent years, non-invasive technologies (which do not require surgical implantation) have been introduced. These new stimulation devices can also stimulate the vagus nerve and help with depression, varying degrees of stress, anxiety, and other nervous disorders. For example, the FDA has approved using the gammaCore in the United States, and the device is also supported in Europe. Another example is the NEMOS system, which stimulates the vagus nerve when applied to the ear.

A more significant proportion of people with epilepsy do not respond to other forms of stimulation. Therefore, this option (electrical stimulation) reduces the likelihood of seizures and other complications associated with low vagal tone. Similarly, people who have been taking medication for depression, anxiety, and stress without results may choose this stimulation method.

Regular stimulation of the vagus nerve keeps it healthy and improves vagal tone. Like muscles, the nerve needs regular exercise to stay toned and function properly. Nutrition and gratitude can improve vagal tone, but there are other ways to stimulate the nerve.

You are not obliged to use all of the methods described below. You can even limit yourself to one or two. There are several options here, but the most important thing is that you stimulate the vagus nerve. This means you should choose activities that you enjoy or that make you feel good. Gradual changes tend to stick better than abrupt, complete lifestyle changes. So start with one or two new things. Then you can build on them gradually.

Improving your lifestyle is an important step, and implementing it could not be so easy. However, don't let this be another resolution you tackle and then drop. It is far too important for that, especially if you suffer from health problems related to vagus nerve dysfunction or damage. You can improve your symptoms, but you have to do the work for this to happen.

Music and binaural beats

Certain types of sound can positively influence the work of the brain. This has been proven for some time, but more and more studies on neuroplasticity and music exist. You may notice that music affects you. It can give you energy or put you in a state of low mood. Some music triggers anger, while other music can calm you down. This is all very important because you can actually use music to improve your vagal tone.

Many people use music to control their moods, but you can further incorporate binaural beats. These are designed to stimulate the brain but are also used to influence the vagus nerve.

Binaural beats are two or more similar sine waves. They must consist of pure tones and usually work best with headphones as they are reproduced in both ears. For example, a pure tone of 500 Hz might be played in one ear while a pure tone of 480 Hz is heard in the other. The result is an auditory illusion that increases the brain's neuroplasticity and makes it more open to memory and learning.

Binaural beats are considered entrainment, where a duo of autonomic rhythmic oscillators works together to interact and synchronize. This technology can influence the body in various ways, including changing heart rate, relaxation, and blood pressure. It is also used to refresh memory and increase concentration.

Often typical music is mixed with binaural beats to make it easier to hear the odd rhythm. You can listen to the music while the binaural beats work with your brain to stimulate it and achieve a higher state of alertness or a more relaxed state. Different beats are used depending on the desired result. They can help you fall asleep, keep you awake without caffeine and even be beneficial in regulating your moods and fighting depression. They all work with the vagus nerve, so Entrainment, in conjunction with the other methods in this book, proves particularly effective in promoting vagal tone.

Even if you don't use binaural beats in your vagal tone routine, you should definitely listen to music. Choose something that you like, and that feels good. You can listen to music on your morning commute to work to improve your mood and increase your tone, or you can listen to it during any break, no matter how short.

Pray

Prayer is not for everyone, but praying to someone or something can also help strengthen the vagus nerve. The act of praying is very similar to meditation and, like meditation, can activate the vagus nerve. When you pray, you concentrate entirely on the prayer. This clears the mind and brings serenity, but it is more than that.

Belief in a more powerful being or force than oneself can provide hope and a sense of security. These are two things that contribute to the well-being of the nervous system.

Visualization

Your mind is a powerful part of your body that is underutilized in terms of improving overall health. Now is an excellent time to start if you have never engaged in visualisation or body awareness. If you like, you can combine this with deep breathing and meditation.

Essentially, close your eyes and imagine your vagus nerve. Please start at the top of your body and imagine it is leading up to your throat. Next, imagine how it helps you to breathe in and out gently. Finally, imagine how the nerve is connected to the different organs. You may not be able to control these organs, but you can imagine them working perfectly.

You can also focus on your heartbeat and try to slow it down consciously. However, it is often enough to become aware of the beat to activate the vagus nerve. Similarly, imagine your digestive system functioning perfectly. This can actually lead to improved function of the gastrointestinal tract.

Focusing on your body and how the vagus nerve works can be very helpful. If you do this regularly for 10 minutes a day, you will notice a surprising improvement in organ function. You may not be able to control your organs consciously, but you can influence their function with your mind.

Practice generosity

Generosity is something that can also stimulate your vagus nerve. It gives you a nice dose of daily interaction with other people and increases your social standing, and it is also a profitable way to feel good about yourself.

Generosity can look like anything that involves giving of yourself. For example, you could provide some change to a beggar, but it is not necessarily about giving money. Other ways to be generous are:

- Give your time: Help someone with housework, sit with someone lonely, or just spend time with someone. For example, you could help out at an older adult's home or just talk to a lonely person in the park. You can make a difference if you get involved in a soup kitchen or a food bank. There are countless ways to volunteer.
- Do you have extra snacks over? Why not give them to someone who needs them? You have the chance to make their day. It's worth taking extra food with you when you go out or to work to share it. It's amazing how much someone's day improves when you give them a chocolate bar or a packet of biscuits.

- Give compliments: Your words can also be kind. Try to give at least five compliments every day. You will feel great, and so will the people who receive them. Look for opportunities to say something nice to others. Don't just focus on the outside; compliment the other person on their inner beauty and make them feel good. Sometimes, a compliment to someone who is always grumpy or in a bad mood can brighten their day.

- Pay for the person sitting in front of you: Pay the bill for someone else at the drive-in or supermarket to sweeten their day and increase your vagal tone at the same time. You never know what someone else is going through, and you could easily change the course of their day as you do your daily business.

- Take in a pet: If you love animals, why not make room in your home for a stray? Then, you can adopt the animal or give it a loving temporary home until it finds its forever home. Pets also have a relaxing effect on people and can provide you with far more than you give the animals. You may even end up in a foster situation where you keep the animal you want to give back later.

- Allow someone to cut in front of you: Allow someone to go in front of you while driving or waiting in line. It costs you no more than a few seconds or a minute, but it is a generous gesture that will lift both spirits. Instead of stirring up anger and frustration, smile, wave the person over, and raise the vagal tone.

All around us are opportunities to be generous. It doesn't have to be a grand gesture, but even small things can help improve the course of someone else's day, including yours. Plus, you have the added benefit of increasing your vagal tone.

Sleeping on the right side

Research is pretty limited in this regard, but anecdotal evidence shows that sleeping on your right side increases vagal tone. So, to be honest, you have nothing to lose by trying it.

Yoga to stimulate the vagus nerve

Yoga is a great way to activate the vagus nerve as it naturally stretches and relaxes the body. In addition, it also allows for mindfulness, which activates the vagus nerve as well. So when you do yoga, you provide a positive attitude and the relaxation you need to encourage your body and mind to slowly let go of the anxiety probably holding you back otherwise.

Just about any posture will help stimulate the vagus nerve, especially if you adopt a position that stretches and relaxes the abdomen. You will have great success if you can use any of these techniques. However, we will look at one pose in particular that is excellent for gentle relaxation. This pose is known as the child's pose and is one of the most basic, beginner-friendly positions you can do in yoga.

Sit with your knees on the floor. They should be slightly apart and toes pressed together behind you. Pull your feet back so that they rest under you and the tops of your feet touch the floor.

Slowly lower your body to the floor. Then, slowly and gently lean forward by placing your hands on the floor and sliding them outwards as you continue to lean forward.

Go as far as you can and stretch slowly and gently as you reach out with your hands. Your hands should reach above your head, and your forehead should rest gently on the floor.

Yoga promotes mental health and balances the vagus nerve network. More and more people are becoming aware of its benefits for the individual's well-being. This has led to a significant increase in yoga classes and centers. The number of students signing up for yoga sessions continues to increase as it is now a beneficial method of controlling the nervous system. When you practice yoga, you will find that you can control your body system better. This is due to its effect on the vagus nerve. Yoga activates the parasympathetic nervous system and improves digestion, function, lung capacity, and blood flow.

Exposure to sunlight

Sun exposure affects our body's cellular functions, which are genetically programmed to depend on how much sunlight we are exposed to. So if you don't spend all day in the sun, whether on the way to work by underground or by car and then come home late at night from work or another activity without enough skin contact with the sun, your cells are less likely to function at their best.

Exposing your eyes and skin to sunlight is important for your circadian rhythm and restful sleep. For example, when light hits your eye (don't look directly at the sun), the melanopsin protein in the retina detects the light with the help of vitamin A and signals to the brain that it is daytime. However, when it gets dark, this signal is switched off. So, according to research, when you expose your eyes and skin to sunlight, your melatonin (sleep hormone) levels increase at night.

Sunlight accelerates serotonin production in the brain and supports the circadian rhythm and the vagus nerve in regulating the heart rate. Therefore, it is recommended to go outside more often on sunny days to feel the sun's warmth.

Chapter 7: What happens when you tone your vagus nerve?

What is a strengthened vagus nerve?

A strengthened vagus nerve is one that operates at peak performance, tirelessly working to keep you and your body secure. When you strengthen your vagus nerve, its efficiency improves significantly, allowing it to function optimally. For instance, if you experience muscle tension, it could also indicate that your vagus nerve is tense. The most effective way to measure the vagus nerve's ability to function optimally is by evaluating its vagal tone through heart rate assessment. The good news is that this process is not complicated at all. A high vagal tone is closely linked to significant heart rate variability during breathing, where the pulse changes slightly over time. Even if your heart rate is around 50 or 60 beats per minute, it's essential to note that the beats are not perfectly separated from each other. Instead, they vary between beats, with one beat occurring a full second apart from the next, while another may be as little as 0.9 seconds apart. These variations are common and are caused by the body's constant changes in regulating the way the heart beats in response to changes. To determine how well your vagus nerve is working, all you need to do is stop and pay attention to your pulse. You don't need to get accurate readings; you just need to make sure that your heart rate changes with your breathing. This is relatively easy if you have a heart rates monitor, such as a Fitbit or other device that records your readings. You can also observe the general trends in your heart rate. For example, if you watch the tracking of your heart rate in real-time, you will most likely notice a difference. You may have a weak vagus nerve if your pulse is steady and does not fluctuate. When you relax, your heart rate slows down, and when your body responds, it speeds up. Remember that your heart rate variability is unique to you as an individual. So pay attention to your trends and don't try to achieve arbitrarily set values. Instead, focus on improving your vagus nerve's strength and efficiency to keep your body healthy and secure.

Toning of the vagus nerve

Toning the vagus nerve does not have to be complicated. In fact, it is straightforward to do at the end of the day. All you have to do is use your vagus nerve more often. However, there is one thing you should not forget: When it comes to strengthening the vagus nerve, it is best to enhance it through use.

Think about it: what do you do when you want to tone your legs? You use them! If you want to tone your abs, you do the same. The training is done through repetitions. This is important to know. You can train your vagus nerve by using it regularly, but if you stop using it at the end of the day, you may find that it loses efficiency over time.

Like all the muscles in your body, the vagus nerve works similarly. You can tense it and build it to its maximum capacity, but the vagus nerve may weaken again if you slack off with exercise. Likewise, your vagus nerve can slowly dwindle and weaken through inactivity, especially if you are in a situation where you no longer use it.

For this reason, the changes you make while reading this manuscript should be considered lifestyle changes - they should be considered long-term changes that you will continue to make regularly. You need to ensure that you are constantly working to keep your vagus nerve in pristine condition so you can rely on it when you need it most.

It is strongly recommended that you approach training the vagus nerve the same way you approach training the muscles. It is important to train regularly to get the best possible results and ensure you get the most out of what you are doing. If you do this, you can ensure your vagus nerve stays in top condition.

The vague tone and its importance

Vagal tone is the activity of the vagus nerve. As we have seen in the previous chapters, the action of the vagus nerve has significant effects on the following:

- Regulation of the heart rate,
- Vasodilation and constriction of the vessels,

- Glandular activity in the heart,
- Glandular activity lung,
- Gastrointestinal sensitivity and motility and
- Regulation of inflammation.

Vagal tone is measured by the consistency of the parasympathetic effect that the vagus nerve exerts in terms of health. While vagal input is consistent, the degree of stimulation it provides is influenced by various factors, including the parasympathetic responses of the autonomic nervous system. This means that vagal tone varies according to the body's internal environment. For example, vagal tone or activity is reduced if the body is stressed.

Vagal tone can diagnose emotional regulation or other factors, such as digestive functions, influenced by parasympathetic responses.

Vagal tone can be measured using either invasive or non-invasive methods. Invasive measurement of vagal tone is characterized by using manual or electrical techniques to stimulate the vagus nerve. In non-invasive methods, vagal tone is usually measured by heart rate and variability. The difference in the time that elapses between heartbeats is called heart rate variability (HRV).

When the vagal tone is high, the heart rate is usually slower, while an increased heart rate indicates that the activity of the vagus nerve is reduced. The vagal tone in the body is a valuable tool for determining emotional, psychological, and even physical disorders that may manifest as a result of inadequate vagal activity or function.

In some people, the vagus nerve activity is healthier and more pronounced than in others, allowing the body to relax quickly after strenuous activity. For example, the stress you feel when you subject your body to a high level of exercise is beneficial, especially when you finish the exercise. As a result, your body gains health and strength, giving you an agreeable mental sense of accomplishment. Another example is the positive feeling you get when you finish a stressful task: "Yes, I did it!" This feeling of accomplishment boosts you when you prepare for the next stressful task because you know you have everything under control.

Please remember that other factors, such as poor lifestyle habits, can also cause low vagal tone, while vagus-friendly habits can increase it. In other words, vagal tone refers to the strength of your vagus response or the degree to which your vagus nerve is active.

It is also worth noting that, according to research in this field, vagal tone is inherited from mother to child. This means mothers who are depressed, anxious, or angry during pregnancy have lower vagal activity. And when their child is born, the newborn has low vagal activity and low levels of dopamine and serotonin.

Vagal tone is the response of the vagus nerve. Among other things, vagal tone is responsible for heart rate, constriction and dilation of blood vessels, glandular activity in the body, and motility.

In general, vagal tone is the baseline for parasympathetic actions. So vagal tone is not always just an indication of whether or not you have a healthy vagus nerve, but you should use it as a good basis for determining what is happening in your body.

That is, we all have the same basic vagal value.

The power of the vagueston

Vagal tone exerts extraordinary power over us. We can have a high or low vagal tone depending on our circumstances. Low vagal tone is familiar in people who are constantly stressed, angry, or anxious. On the other hand, those who are always happy, cheerful, and optimistic have a high vagal tone. Some parents, especially first-time mothers, may experience high-stress levels, restless sleep, and anxiety. Your vagal tone will improve if you are positive, optimistic, and in good physical and mental health. It is amazing what vagal tone can do for you and the results it can achieve.

Our serotonin and dopamine levels are also influenced by vagal tone. When it is high, serotonin and dopamine levels increase; when vagal tone is low, serotonin and dopamine levels decrease.

Your vagal tone regulates your heart rate and can predict the condition of your heart, breathing, and physical health. High vagal tone is associated with increased heart rate variability. Lower heart rate variability, on the other hand, corresponds to low it.

Understanding how your vagal tone works and its importance can help you solve many problems. Understanding this can help you overcome symptoms such as depression, anxiety, and stress.

Remember that your vagal tone affects everything from heart rate to breathing to physical and mental ailments. By gaining control over it, you can avert the development of these problems.

If you find that your vagal tone is not high, you don't have to worry. There are ways to increase it through stimulation. For example, if you suffer from a treatment-resistant condition like depression, you can use a device to stimulate the vagus nerve, which we will discuss later. But we will also give you uncomplicated solutions for stimulating your vagus nerve and thus stimulating your vagal tone.

Measurement of vagal tone

Invasive and non-invasive methods can measure vagal tone. Some people receive manual or electrical stimulation of the vagus nerve, which we will discuss in more detail later.

Usually, vagal tone is measured with non-invasive methods for obvious reasons. However, in most cases, it is measured through the heart rate. Remember that a few chapters ago, we talked about the internal pacemaker that we all have. A healthy heart naturally generates electrical activity and sends impulses to the rest of the body, independent of any other vagus nerve stimulation.

This electrical activity sets the beat of the heart. The beats per minute (BPM) of an average person with a healthy heart are between 60 and 100.

If the BPM is too high, it is probably slowed down by the autonomic nervous system; if it is too low, it is increased. These electrical energies stimulate the heart. At the same time, the autonomic nervous system works to check the heart rate.

Vagal tone is measured when you track your heart and breathing rates. Your heart rate increases when you inhale and decreases when you exhale. The difference between your heart rate when you breathe in and your heart rate when you breathe out is your vagal tone. So to determine whether your vagal tone is low or high, you would first need to measure the time variation (in milliseconds) between successive heartbeats, called heart rate variability (HRV) - a golden standard for measuring the strength of vagal tone.

Heart rate is essentially controlled by these two components, natural electrical activity and the autonomic nervous system, which together balance the overall system and keep your heart beating at a regular rhythm.

The other area that vagal tone measures are your breathing. Breathing is the cause of fluctuations in heart rate. Remember: when you breathe in, your heart rate increases; when you breathe out, it decreases. This is a natural process that occurs not only in humans but also in animals. As we get older, the vagal tone tends to decrease. However, adults with good heart health will continue to have higher vagal tone than those with poorer health. An excellent example of this is professional athletes. Because of their training, they are able to control their heart rate, which in turn affects the control of their vagal tone. On the other hand, people prone to diabetes or other similar diseases or conditions will notice that their heart health is not optimal, so their vagal tone will be lower.

Knowing this data can provide information on the behavior and functioning of the heart. Vagal tone and heart health can be measured to determine any diseases, conditions or disorders. Adequate vagal tone essentially signals that all is well and that heart rate, breathing, and the like are functioning correctly.

Vagal tone, as we have already learned, can also inform us about things in our body that we may not otherwise be able to recognize. For example, it can inform us about how we react to certain triggers that may directly result from certain anxiety disorders or depression. Any effect that seems abnormal or does not match what we are used to feeling can be the proximate cause of low vagal tone.

High Vaguston

The strength of the vagal tone determines how well the body functions. High vagal tone supports the body's systems, such as regulating blood sugar levels, reducing the risk of diabetes, stroke, cardiovascular disease and migraines, and improving digestion. High vagal tone is also associated with elevated mood, increased resistance to stress, and reduced anxiety. In addition, high vagal tone indicates high heart rate variability (more on this in the next section).

Low Vaguston

Low vagal tone means that the vagus nerve response is low. Low vagal tone can lead to a variety of health problems, including cardiovascular disease, stroke, diabetes, depression, negative moods, chronic fatigue, and an increased risk of being affected by inflammatory conditions such as autoimmune diseases (rheumatoid arthritis, inflammatory bowel disease, and more). In addition, low vagal tone indicates low heart rate variability.

According to one study, people with inflammatory diseases often have low heart rate variability, which can trigger the release of pro-inflammatory cytokines, leading to increased sympathetic nervous system activity and stress hormones.

Check your heart rate variability

Heart rate variability can be traced back to our autonomic nervous system, which is divided into the sympathetic (fight or flight) and parasympathetic (rest and digest) nervous systems and is partly responsible for regulating essential body systems such as heart rate, respiration, blood pressure, and digestion. Therefore, heart rate variability indicates that both nervous systems are functioning.

Intrinsic heart rate measures a state in which neither the parasympathetic nor the sympathetic nervous system is regulating. When the intrinsic heart rate is not subject to autonomic regulation, a healthy heart beats in the range of 60-100 beats per minute.

The parasympathetic nervous system regulates the heart rate by lowering it from its intrinsic level while providing variability between successive heartbeats. Parasympathetic regulation almost immediately affects a few heartbeats at a time, after which the heart rate returns to its intrinsic level. Sympathetic regulation, on the other hand, increases the heart rate beyond its natural rate, leaving little or no room for variability between heartbeats. Sympathetic nervous system regulation affects a few consecutive heartbeats.

The result is that the heart rate is lower in the resting and digesting state, but the HRV is higher, while in the fight and flight state the heart rate is higher, but the HRV is lower.

Even at rest, circumstances such as stress can cause the parasympathetic nervous system to be deactivated while the sympathetic nervous system is activated.

According to research, people with high HRV have better cardiovascular fitness. In addition, they are less sensitive to stress, while those with low HRV suffer from conditions such as depression, anxiety, and cardiovascular disease.

In general, HRV can provide feedback on your lifestyle, which is a good way to determine how your nervous system is responding to your feelings, thoughts, and emotions, as well as to the environment.

Healthy irregularities accompany a healthy heartbeat. If your heart rate is 60 beats per minute, it does not mean it beats once every second. The time between your heartbeats may differ. For example, the interval between two consecutive heartbeats may be 0.5 ms, and between two other consecutive beats, it may be 1.5 ms. Even if the interval is measured in fractions of a second, you can feel the difference.

To find out your HRV, take your pulse by placing two fingers on your carotid artery (on the side of your neck) or your wrist, and then take a deep breath in and out. When you exhale, the interval between heartbeats becomes longer (the heart rate decreases); when you inhale, it becomes shorter (the heart rate increases). Note that physical activity can affect HRV, resulting in a more even interval between beats. However, a high interval between inhalation and exhalation at rest indicates high HRV - a good sign of stress management and good vagal tone (high vagal tone).

On the other hand, if you have a trivial temporal fluctuation between inhalation and exhalation at rest, this indicates low HRV, which is usually a fight-or-flight response to stress and implies a low vagal tone, which means you are unable to cope with stress. If you remain in this state of low vagal tone for a prolonged period of time, you risk poor performance and health.

Measuring HRV from your pulse gives you a rough idea of your HRV. However, it does not provide an accurate HRV measurement because it is difficult to perceive variations in heartbeats without special technology. The technology you choose to use will determine how you calculate your HRV.

The electrocardiogram (ECG) machine is a commonly used technology today. This device records the electrical impulse generated by the contraction of your heart. The data obtained can be used to calculate your HRV. Measuring HRV with ECG technology usually required a visit to a doctor, where complex equipment and electrodes were attached to the body. However, thanks to technological advances, this can now be done in the comfort of your home with heart rate monitors such as the Polar H7 heart rate strap.

A wearable smartwatch with an integrated ECG device has also been shown in research to be a reliable method of measuring HRV. The FDA has approved the Apple Watch, for example. This allows users of the Apple Watch to determine their HRV while on the go easily. Another technology that does not use the ECG to measure HRV but requires an optical sensor to measure heartbeat intervals is photoplethysmography (PPG). PPG uses a light source and a photodetector on the skin's surface to detect changes in blood volume. For example, the well-known Oura ring uses PPG technology to determine HRV.

The good thing about such devices is that they are non-invasive and can therefore be worn on the wrist, finger, or around the chest to measure HRV even during sleep - this is highly recommended because the more detailed the measurement is taken at rest and without distraction, the more reliable the data.

Interpretation of heart rate variability results

There is no standard procedure for the best possible HRV values, which is quite understandable considering that there are different methods for recording and calculating HRV.

According to a 2016 Health and Quality of Life Outcomes, a study published in Sports Medicine Research, low HRV values are <780 ms, and high HRV values are >=780 ms. HRV tends to be high when a person is healthy and fit, and how high it can depend on the person.

Since a number of factors such as age, gender, body functions, lifestyle, and even hormones can influence HRV readings, it is advisable that you do not compare your HRV reading with that of other people (even those of the same gender). Instead, it would be best to focus on your HRV and its trends. For example, suppose you use trends to compare your daily HRV readings. In that case, you should take the measurement using the same technology and under analog conditions - preferably at night when you are asleep, as this is when your body is resting.

It can be said that you have a low HRV when the intervals of your heartbeat are constantly low and a high HRV when the intervals are constantly high.

Increase your vagal tone

Increased vagal tone activates the parasympathetic nervous system, which helps the body to relax more quickly after stress, regulate mood and cope better with anxiety.

To some extent, the strength of your vagal tone is genetic, just like the mother who passed on her low vagal tone to her unborn child during pregnancy. However, this does not mean low vagal tone cannot be altered or increased. Vagal tone can be increased through a number of methods, including some recommended natural exercises and practices, such as deep breathing, as well as the use of electrical stimulation techniques.

Chapter 8: Diaphragmatic Breathing and Slow Exhalation

When you use diaphragmatic breathing, you are trying to relax your body. This type of breathing can reduce your stress and heart rate and allows you to regulate the stimulation of your vagus nerve. With diaphragmatic breathing, you perform breathing exercises that directly target the diaphragm, the muscle in your abdomen that controls your breathing.

Find a place where you feel comfortable to start this process. Start sitting, standing, or lying down in a position that is comfortable for you. For example, you can stretch out on the floor or a bed or sit in a comfortable chair. Relax your shoulders once you have found the most comfortable position.

Place one hand on your chest and the other on your belly while your shoulders relax. Inhale through your nose for about two seconds and notice how the air expands your abdomen. Make sure your chest remains still as you breathe in - this way, you know you are breathing through the diaphragm and not through the chest, through which the breathing will not be as deep and relaxing.

Press on your belly to remind yourself to exhale with it and exhale for two seconds with your lips pressed together as if you were trying to take a sip from a straw or water bottle. Repeat this process several times, gradually increasing the time for inhaling and exhaling to five seconds each. This way, you slow your breathing to six breaths per minute, which is ideal for activating the vagus nerve.

How-To: Diaphragmatic Breathing

There are several ways to train diaphragmatic breathing. The primary purpose of this type of breathing is to focus on the diaphragm. Some people like to practice this type of breathing during meditation, which has its benefits.

When practicing diaphragmatic breathing, it is crucial to follow the steps below. First, make sure you have a straight posture. This is a significant part of the exercise. Regardless of how you sit, use your body as little as possible. This not only helps to minimize pain but also prevents other injuries from occurring. Most people like to sit where they can feel themselves straightening and stretching. As you inhale, you stretch upwards, and as you exhale, you relax your body. The perfect place for this exercise is a chair. Avoid beds or sofas, as they can lead to incorrect posture.

When inhaling, ensure you inhale from the lungs and the whole body. Breathing in with the whole body creates a feeling of grounding. You will find that a more robust grounding helps to stabilize your state, makes you more aware, and thus makes you much happier.

When you inhale, you should notice the movement of your diaphragm. When you do this, you will see that your blood pressure and heart rate variability change, and you will feel better.

You can thank the vagus nerve for that.

So when you breathe from your diaphragm, it's not just a temporary means to improve your health; it touches all fronts and makes you feel good, happy, and at ease.

Once you have practiced this form of breathing, you will notice improvements directly. You may see that your anxious stomach feeling has disappeared, that you are more relaxed than before, or that you feel sexually freer and less stressed. You will be more aware of your body and its well-being after practicing this type of breathing.

What happens when you breathe through your diaphragm?

Diaphragmatic breathing is one of the most recognized ways to stimulate the vagus nerve, reduce the body's sympathetic activity, and promote parasympathetic activity, i.e., reduce stress and relaxation.

When you practice diaphragmatic breathing, you trigger the release of acetylcholine, which helps to reduce stress in the body, lower the heart rate, slow down breathing, tame the inflammatory system, and send out neurotransmitters that prevent further inflammation. Diaphragmatic breathing also plays a significant role in our inner peace. You will find that you can better control your emotions, your psychological adjustments, and how you express yourself emotionally. You may even notice that you react more empathetically to different stimuli.

You will find that when you pay attention to your breathing and well-being, you also feel good about yourself and your surroundings. Doing this exercise for 15 minutes daily, being more reflective, or following a guided meditation can help reduce stress and promote a more mindful experience between you and your body.

Diaphragmatic breathing and meditation

As already mentioned, diaphragmatic breathing is a form of meditation. One of my favorite meditation techniques is to inhale for five seconds and then exhale for ten seconds. When you inhale, your heart rate increases, and when you exhale, it decreases. This kind of breathing can promote both body stability and attention.

Some people do this kind of breathing before they meditate. It will help you get into the correct state of mind.

I like to do these breathing exercises while a guided meditation plays in the background. I concentrate on my breathing while the guided meditation is playing. I allow myself to become fully aware of the present moment.

Let's say I listen to a guided meditation about giving thanks to the environment and expressing my gratitude. I will find that I feel better and am happier if I breathe deeply and mindfully beforehand.

You don't have to meditate to practice diaphragmatic breathing, but combining it with meditation offers a more meaningful and grounded experience.

Most people are not aware that diaphragmatic breathing is a form of grounding. So if you don't use diaphragmatic breathing for meditation and want to come down, sit down and breathe from your diaphragm for 5-10 minutes. After that, do something that doesn't tire the mind, such as sleeping or listening to relaxing music. This is a great way to stimulate the vagus nerve, and if you breathe from the diaphragm while doing this, you will find that you are much more in tune with your body and well-being.

Deep breathing is beneficial because it helps you focus during meditation, but it also helps loosen and energize your body. It also helps to clear the mind. For example, if you practice deep diaphragmatic breathing before meditation, you can stimulate the neural pathways, which leads to a much better, more relaxed state of mind during meditation.

Think about how constant your attention is throughout the day. Perhaps this is why you cannot relax or activate the vagus nerve. When you use the vagus nerve, you intentionally direct and control the amount of your attention. You choose what to focus on when you wilfully direct and maintain your attention.

Practicing diaphragmatic breathing helps you relax your body and figure out what you need to get done, whether during the day or throughout the week. It can also improve your problem-solving skills, mental clarity, and overall mental health and awareness.

As mentioned earlier, diaphragmatic breathing also helps to clear your head. When you breathe deeply, your brain is better supplied with blood, which increases your alertness.

The importance of proper breathing

Breathing is the most mundane action for most people. You don't have to worry about life because breathing goes on. Even if it is unconscious, you can control your breathing, which significantly affects how your body functions.

Without delving too deeply into human anatomy, it is important to know that breathing is achieved through one large dome-shaped muscle, the diaphragm, and many smaller muscles called the intercostal muscles. The chest and internal cavity can open and contract as these muscles contract and relax, allowing the muscles to expand or contract alternately, naturally, or actively. Without your knowledge, your heart continues to beat, and many of your digestive system's muscles function the same way. With the help of the skeletal muscles, you can control your movements as you wish.

However, breathing can be both conscious and unconscious. For example, you can consciously take a deep breath and "suck in only a little air" or exhale as gently or quickly as possible.

You can also control other aspects of your life by controlling your breathing. For example, when you slow your breathing, your heart rate gradually increases while breathing rises rapidly. In other words, you can become excited when you breathe steadily and quickly. The capacity of your brain, metabolism, and virtually all other factors influence the speed, length, and rhythm of your breathing and the different oxygen intake. The amount of oxygen you take in with each inhalation is determined by your body, but you can control your oxygen consumption to a certain extent.

Apart from the ability to control breathing, your daily life also benefits from its biological and physiological importance in many ways. For example, breathing is an excellent starting point for concentration. Breathing is always there, easy to observe, and can quickly become your priority.

Breathing techniques play an essential role in meditation practice. Many types of meditation, such as Zen meditation, rely almost exclusively on breathing and focus on breathing, while all other forms of meditation would benefit greatly from proper breathing.

There are apparent benefits to eliciting a desired calming response: you can change your heartbeat and arouse or calm yourself through the breath alone. Even if you cannot control your body during certain meditation sessions, it will obviously help to calm your mind.

Regrettably, most of you will spend your lives not paying attention to your breathing, partly because you do not know how to breathe correctly, thinking that breathing just happens. But breathing is much more than just a feature of the body, as it can be the key to your well-being and enhance your meditation practice.

Breathing exercises have various health benefits through increased and more effective oxygen uptake and improved use of the abdominal muscles, even when done just for themselves. Most of the strategies mentioned in this book consciously engage the abdominal wall. Not only does this serve to stimulate the often sluggish abdominal muscles, develop increasingly better, more natural posture and relieve much of the pressure on the spine that sometimes causes lower back pain, but the deep muscles will also function and become more assertive if the abdomen is constantly emptied and actively used along with other often active muscles.

Diaphragmatic breathing techniques

You can try to relieve the symptoms and feel better if you feel breathless with pain. Let's go through some things you can do at any time of the day or that you can do yourself over a more extended period.

1. Lengthen your exhalation

You can't always relax by simply breathing in. This is because deep breaths are connected to the sympathetic nervous system, which controls the fight or flight response. On the other hand, breathing out is connected to the parasympathetic nervous system, which inhibits our body's ability to calm down.

Excessive deep breathing can lead to hyperventilation. Hyperventilation reduces the amount of oxygen-rich blood flowing to your brain. When anxious or stressed, we breathe too deeply more easily and hyperventilate - even if we want to do the opposite.

Before taking a deep breath, first exhale completely. Drive the oxygen out of your body and let your lungs do their job by breathing in air. First, try to exhale a little more than you inhale. Breathe out for six seconds and then in for four seconds. This exercise should take about two to five minutes.

2. Abdominal breathing

Diaphragmatic breathing (the muscle located under the lungs) can help reduce the amount of breathing the body has to do. Learn how the diaphragm breathes:

Inhale
- Lie on the floor or a mattress with a pillow under your head and knees to get comfortable. Or sit on a comfortable chair, relax your head, neck, and shoulders, and bend your knees.
- Place your hand under your chest and the other on your heart.
- Breathe in and out with your nose and notice how or if you breathe and move your belly and chest.
- Should one separate the breath so that the air gets into the lungs? And the opposite? Could you breathe because your heart beats in your belly?

After all, the chest should not move when you breathe, but the abdomen.

Practice abdominal breathing:

- Sit or lie down as described above.
- Place one hand on the neck and the other on the upper abdomen.
- Breathe in through your nose and feel your belly rise. Your chest remains pretty still.
- Close your lips and exhale through your mouth. Try to push the air out at the end of the breath using the abdominal muscles.

You need to practice it daily so that this type of breathing becomes automatic. Try to practice three to four times a day for up to 10 minutes. It may feel laborious if you have not used your diaphragm to breathe before. However, with practice, it will become easier.

3. Breath focus

Deep, concentrated, and slow breathing can help to reduce anxiety. This technique can be done sitting or lying in a quiet, comfortable place. Then follow the steps below:

- Notice how you normally breathe in and out. Mentally scan your body. You may feel tensions in your body that you have never felt before.
- Breathe in slowly and deeply through your nose.
- Notice how your belly and upper body have expanded.
- Breathe out in a way that feels comfortable and sigh if necessary.
- Concentrate on raising and lowering your belly for a few minutes.
- Choose a word that you focus on and vocalize as you exhale. Words like "safety" and "relaxation" can be adequate.
- Imagine the air you breathe in as a gentle wave washing over you.
- Visualize your exhalation driving out negative, worrying thoughts and energy.
- When you are upset, pay attention to your breath and breathe softly.

If possible, use this method for up to 20 minutes per day.

4. Breathing evenly

Another form of breathing from ancient pranayama yoga is even breathing. A workshop and a lying posture will help you practice even breathing. Regardless of your position, make sure you are comfortable.

- Close your eyes and notice how many breaths you usually inhale.
- Then count slowly 1-2-3-4 while inhaling with your nose.
- Breathe out in the same way for four seconds.
- Notice your body's sensations of fullness and absence as you breathe in and out.

If you continue to practice even breathing, the second count may be different. Keep the inhalation and exhalation in the same way.

5. Resonance breathing

Resonant breathing, also known as coherent breathing, helps you to overcome your fears and relax. Please try it out:

- Close your eyes and lie down.
- Breathe gently through your nose, keep your mouth closed, and count for six seconds.
- Do not overfill your lungs with oxygen.
- Breathe for six seconds and let the air escape slowly and easily from your body. Please do not force it.
- Continue for up to 10 minutes.
- Make sure you have a few minutes left and focus on the sensations of your body.

6. The Breath of the Lion

The breath of the lion stands for a particularly powerful exhalation.

- Find a comfortable place to kneel, cross your knees, and combine your legs to exert the lion's breath. If this position is uncomfortable, sit cross-legged.
- Stretch the legs and feet to the thighs and pull the palms outwards.
- Breathe deeply through your nose.
- Breathe out through your nose and let it say "ha."
- Breathe by opening your mouth as wide as possible and sticking your tongue to your ear as far as possible.
- When breathing, concentrate on the center of the forehead (third eye) or the tip of the nose.
- Keep your mouth quiet when you breathe in again.
- Repeat up to six times and change the ankle crucible when you are halfway through the stage.

7. Alternate breathing with the nostril

Sit in a comfortable place and try to repeat the nasal breathing, stretch your spine and open your chest. Place your left hand and raise your right hand. Then place your right hand's upper and middle fingers on your forehead between your eyebrows. Breathe in and out.

Close your right nose with your right thumb and inhale slowly with your left nose.

- Pinch the nose between the left and right thumbs and hold your breath for one second.
- Close your left nose with your finger on the right ring, exhale, and wait a moment before inhaling again.
- Breathe in slowly through the right nostril.
- Close your eyes again for a second, and hold inside.
- Then open your eyes and exhale on the left side before inhaling again.
- Repeat this inhalation and exhalation process up to 10 times through one of the two nostrils. Each pass should take up to 40 seconds.

8. Valsalva maneuver

This technique can help you understand how your heart works, especially the autonomic nervous system. If you use this method, remember that those with heart problems should consult a doctor before trying this procedure. It strains the heart but also causes the heart rate to be controlled.
This method is mainly used when your heart rate is excessively high, such as during a panic attack. When used correctly, your body will regulate itself so that you can slow down your breathing and regulate yourself better. The procedure consists of four phases followed by five steps.
These five steps take you through four different physiological phases that can effectively manage your body. You will feel better and more balanced as you go through each of these phases. These phases are:

- ***Phase 1:*** You create pressure in your chest by blowing against the closed airways while supporting yourself downwards. This forces the blood into the limbs, causing a sharp rise in blood pressure.
- ***Phase 2:*** They cause your blood pressure to drop as blood flows from the veins back to the heart. The autonomic nervous system senses this drop and increases the heart rate in response, causing the blood pressure to return to the healthy range.
- ***Phase 3:*** You relax and release the breath and the pressure you have created. This causes the blood pressure to drop again.
- ***Phase 4:*** As the blood returns to the heart, blood flow returns to normal, but blood pressure rises in response to the constricted blood vessels, and the blood pressure causes the heart rate to regulate as well.
- ***Breathe deeply and slowly.***

Since the vagus nerve is controlled by a series of parasympathetic nerve impulses, better control and coordination of this nerve is possible. This can be achieved by practicing deep and slow breathing techniques. This can be very useful when the body is in a state of anxiety and stress. You can take a few minutes and consciously slow down the speed at which you inhale. The inhalation and exhalation of air are done through the diaphragm. You should notice your belly moving up and down. If you do this for a more extended period of time, your vagus nerve will be stimulated. This practice increases the speed at which the vagus nerve sends impulses to the brain and back to the different parts of the body.
To begin diaphragmatic breathing, do the following:
Either sit on a chair and support your head, neck, and shoulders against the back of the chair, or lie on your back on the floor or bed, supporting your head and feet with a pillow.
Place one hand on your chest and the other on your stomach.
Close your eyes and breathe slowly and deeply through your nose into your belly (i.e., expand your diaphragm) until you count to five, then pause.
Breathe out slowly through the mouth, counting to ten.
Repeat the same process for about 5-10 minutes

What happens when you stimulate your vagus nerve with diaphragmatic breathing?

Diaphragmatic breathing is not only good for you because it stimulates the body and blood flow. It can also help alleviate oxidative stress and provide natural antioxidants to the body. In addition, this type of breathing can help with aging, cancer prevention, and autoimmune diseases. It also helps increase melatonin levels, contributing to better sleep and overall happiness.

It can help improve the body's defense mechanisms against other oxidants and protect you from free radicals, which can directly impact your aging and well-being.

Your insulin level also increases, which reduces the risk of developing diabetes. Diaphragmatic breathing also reduces blood sugar levels in the body and reactive metabolites. Diaphragmatic breathing improves your lung functions and strengthens your heart and breathing.

Apart from these effects, diaphragmatic breathing also reduces stress, anxiety, and depression and improves your emotions by allowing you to control them.

Chapter 9: Why it is important to have healthy gut bacteria

The number of genes in the microbiota of an organism is more than 200 times the number of genes in the human genome. The microbiome can weigh up to 2.5 kilograms.

The microbiome is crucial for human development, immunity, and nutrition. Bacteria that live inside us are not invaders but rather beneficial colonizers. Infection-causing microbes evolve over time and alter gene expression and metabolic processes, resulting in an unusual immune response to chemicals and tissues usually found in the body. Experience shows that autoimmune diseases are not passed on through DNA inheritance in the family but through the body's microbiome. A few examples: The gut microbiome differs like an overweight twin and a slim twin. Overweight twins have lower bacterial diversity and higher enzyme rates, which means they digest food and produce calories more efficiently. Obesity has also been linked to an imbalance of bacteria in the stomach.

Type I diabetes is an autoimmune disease associated with an unstable gut microbiome. In animal studies, bacteria play a crucial role in the development of diabetes.

House dust from dogs can reduce the immune response to allergens and other asthma triggers by changing the composition of the gut microbiome. Children living in households with pets are less likely to develop allergies.

What is the Human Microbiome Project (HMP)?

The human microbiome is being mapped in global scientific projects, providing insights into previously unknown species and genomes. Another project funded by the National Human Genome Research Institute (NHGRI), part of the National Institutes of Health (NIH), is the Human Microbiome Project (HMP). The HMP was started in 2008 as an extension of the Human Genome Project. It is a five-year, $150 million feasibility study being conducted at a number of centers in the United States.

The HMP aims to study humans as a supraorganism composed of non-human and human cells to describe the human microbiome and investigate its role in human health and disease.

The main objective of the HMP is to classify the metagenome (the set of genomes of all microbes) of 300 healthy people over time—a sample of five body regions: Hair, mouth, nose, stomach, and vagina.

Why is the human microbiome important?

A person's microbiome can influence their susceptibility to infectious diseases and contribute to chronic digestive systems diseases such as Crohn's disease and irritable bowel syndrome. Many microbiota collections reinforce how a patient responds to drug therapy. A mother's microbiota can have an impact on the health of her children. Scientists studying the human microbiome are discovering previously unknown bacteria and genes. Genetic studies assessing the relative abundance of different species in the human microbiome have linked certain combinations of microbial species to specific aspects of human health. With a better understanding of the diversity of microbes in the human microbiome, new treatments can be developed, such as adding more "healthy" bacteria to alleviate a bacterial infection brought on by a "bad" bacterium. The HMP serves as a guide to define the role of the microbiome in health, nutrition, immunity and disease.

Afferent vagus nerves control food intake in the gastrointestinal tract. However, in obesity, the vagal responses of the gastrointestinal tract to enhancement are different, resulting in a shift away from satiety and towards increased food intake. Ten vagal pathways that do not function properly are involved in the progression of obesity and the failure to lose weight.

Numerous studies have shown that gut microbiota is linked to weight maintenance. The gut microbiota favors the production of short-chain unsaturated fats (SCFAs), which produce substances that can act on the vagal afferent nerves to increase the feeling of satiety. In particular, butyrate can directly activate the vagal afferent nerves in the small intestine.

Gut hormones activate vagal afferent neurons, the crucial neural pathway through which data about ingested supplements reach the focal sensory system (CNS) and play a role in GI capacity and satiety. Vagal afferent neurons can even become resistant to the hormone leptin, which controls the feeling of hunger.

In a rat model, a high-fat diet led to changes in the gut microbiota, and this imbalance caused gut irritation and a "faulty gut." In addition, the infiltration of toxins into the bloodstream led to changes in the capacity of vagal neurons.

Another advantageous position of the vagus nerve is that it can reduce the aggravation that occurs when a person gains weight. The vagus nerve can also minimize insulin resistance. Experts advised rodents to follow either a high-fat or high-fat diet combined with vagus nerve stimulation. The rodents that received only a high-fat diet developed several adverse effects in the brain, including insulin resistance, oxidative stress, irritation, and the death of cells known as apoptosis, all leading to cognitive decline.

In any case, the group that ate a high-fat diet at the same time as stimulating the vagus nerve showed an improvement in infractions and insulin sensitivity of the cerebrum and decimated mitochondrial destruction of the brain as well as cell apoptosis. In addition, stimulation of the vagus nerve improved intellectual abilities.

On the other hand, an overly dynamic vagus nerve may also play a role in bulimia nervosa. An increase in vagal afferent movement is associated with overeating and retching in this disorder. Inhibition of vagal afferent activity in patients with extreme bulimia nervosa results in a rapid and tangible decrease in binge eating and vomiting as opposed to controls and a reduction of bothersome symptoms.

Balancing the gut microbiome to heal the vagus nerve

Remember that the gut and the vagus nerve are closely connected - we have studied this many times. So this means that you should also be able to heal the vagus nerve and your parasympathetic response through the gut. You often see this with people trying to treat mental health problems - they often change their diet to something healthier to ensure they are as healthy and effective as possible. Finally, the gut communicates with the brain, so much so that it is often referred to as the second brain. Your gut controls your behavior thanks to the bacteria in this system.

Plant-based diet

A plant-based diet is central - it provides a lot of fiber, which helps regulate the digestive system. This food passes through the system completely undigested until it reaches the large intestine, where bacteria begin to break it down. They can break down much of the fiber through fermentation and the release of polysaccharides. In the process, they convert them into fatty acids used for energy. This process helps the cells in your colon and provides them with the energy they need to keep the whole system running effectively.
Of course, it is also important to remember that fiber keeps all the food in your body moving. So with enough fiber, problems with constipation or diarrhea should stop.

Fermented food

Fermented foods may have an intense, unpleasant taste at first, but if you can get a taste for them, they are especially beneficial to your health. They contain all kinds of bacteria that are useful for your gut. The more healthy bacteria there are, the less room there is for harmful, unhealthy bacteria to cause you problems in the long run. So if you try to eat some of these fermented foods, you should be able to restore your gut balance.
When it comes to fermented foods, try to eat them at least once a day, better twice. Some people prefer tempeh or miso, others kimchi for a quick, spicy bite, and others prefer a scoop of sauerkraut on a sausage. Whatever your taste preferences, spicy, savory, or otherwise, there should be something for you.

Polyphenol

Polyphenol is a micronutrient that acts as an antioxidant. When you take antioxidants, you can inhibit inflammation in the body, which allows for the healing and treatment of several diseases discussed in this book. The antioxidant properties also ensure that the beneficial bacteria thrive while eliminating the harmful bacteria that will only cause problems in the future.

You can find polyphenols in various foods that you may even be excited to see are proven to heal your gut biome: Dark chocolate and red wine are two fantastic sources high in polyphenols. Other sources include blueberries, cherries, and green tea. Of course, you want to up the antioxidants.

Prebiotics

Foods rich in prebiotics essentially feed the good bacteria in your gut. Prebiotics are fibers that you can't digest, but bacteria can. So if you flood your body with these prebiotics by eating them regularly, you will find that your body will be better able to maintain the balance of good bacteria you need.

Some foods are rich in these prebiotics, such as bananas that are not yet ripe, oatmeal, rice, or potatoes that have been cooked and then cooled to allow the starch to settle back down onions and garlic. Your breath and friends may not thank you for eating your daily dose of garlic and onions, but your gut bacteria will be thrilled.

Probiotics

In addition to the prebiotics you take, you should also use a probiotic. By taking probiotics, you can effectively grow the bacteria needed to support the good gut bacteria in your digestive tract. When you take them, you are reintroducing these helpful bacteria into your gut, laying the groundwork for them to thrive and take over so that you can effectively heal your gut.

When buying probiotics, make sure they are high in Lactobacillus and Bifidobacterium. Especially those that belong to the class of soil-based organisms. They are more likely to survive the digestive process alive and develop normally. You should also ensure that your chosen source has a high diversity.

Limit sugar

You are not doing yourself any favors with sugar. The harmful bacteria are the only bacteria happy about artificial and added refined sugar. Of course, these bacteria also want to convince you that you need more of it to get through the day, causing you to crave sugary foods while feeling miserable at the same time. It is much better to avoid added sugar altogether.

Beware of antibiotics

Of course, you can't do without antibiotics completely. However, they can sometimes be helpful, especially if you are ill or have an infection. If this is the case, try to be proactive to preserve as much of your beneficial gut flora as possible. If you are taking antibiotics, try taking them along with antibiotic-resistant yeast and prebiotics, and probiotics. The hope is that the good bacteria will continue to populate the gut, even though they may be wiped out with each dose of antibiotics you take. In addition, protecting the gut and enriching it with good bacteria between antibiotic doses can alleviate some of the stress and discomfort that comes with the death of gut bacteria, such as diarrhea and nausea.

Chronic inflammation of the intestine

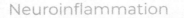

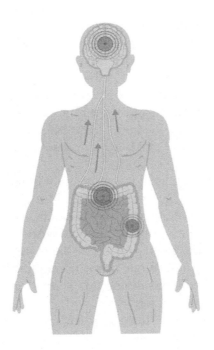

The white blood cells can become desensitized to inflammation if it is constant over a long time. These white blood cells are the body's little soldiers. They protect it. Ongoing inflammation has a negative effect on them.

Inflammations in the intestines are tricky because we cannot easily perceive the symptoms. They only manifest themselves when the situation becomes grave. You can find a test online or see your doctor. The most common cause of intestinal inflammation is an imbalance in the microbiome population of the digestive tract. There are other causes, such as eating inflammatory foods, but the one mentioned above is the most common.

Not only white blood cells and antibodies can become desensitized to inflammation. Constant inflammation can also cause the vagus nerve to wear itself out. It begins to learn to ignore inflammatory signals, which leads to a catastrophic situation because it no longer does its job of sending signals to the antibodies to inhibit inflammation. If it does not do its job, the inflammation continues, and the antibodies start attacking healthy cells in the body.

Young people are relatively safe, but after the age of 30, inflammation decreases. The functionality of the vagus nerve and vagal tone have decreased significantly. Over time, it has learned to ignore inflammation symptoms and signals. Not only does age reduce the influence of the vagus nerve and vagal tone on inflammation, but other factors that put people in a vulnerable health situation can also contribute. Pregnancy and childbirth are examples, but also illness and emotional trauma.

Gluten is another issue related to gut health. Gluten is a component of wheat, and while it is a trigger for people with coeliac disease, more and more people are choosing gluten-free products because it affects gut health. Gluten often does not contribute to a healthy gut but rather an overgrowth of bacteria. Therefore, it may be beneficial for you to reduce or eliminate gluten. While this is not an immediate problem for most people, it is worth considering unless they have coeliac disease. Then, it can't hurt to give it a try.

Gluten is one of the prime suspects when searching for the culprit that prevents your vagus nerve from being adequately stimulated. The Western diet contains a lot of gluten in the form of bread, cereals, and wheat products. Sugars, including gluten, are abundant in our bodies. Consumption of gluten causes debauched inflammation in the body. If the vagus nerve is not adequately stimulated, this can lead to problems with the microbiome and the inability to fight inflammation.

Nowadays, there are many gluten-free alternatives. Those who have coeliac disease or chronic intestinal inflammation can benefit significantly from these alternatives. Rice, oat, soy, and other alternatives are among them. Find out about gluten-free products that can replace your current foods.

In your diet, also pay attention to what other foods you eat. Eliminate all other toxic foods from your diet, such as processed foods. You should also try to cut sugar out of your diet or at least reduce it. Overeating sugar in a single day contributes to the poisoning of the body and our vagus nerve, so be sure to work on eliminating it.

A natural and healthy diet is most likely the best thing you can do. Also, avoid taking too many antibiotics as this can affect your gut health, affecting the vagus nerve.

Your gut is connected to your vagus nerve, believe it or not. In this chapter, we have described some essential aspects of the connection between the vagus nerve and gut health and how to care for it.

Chapter 10: The benefits of vagus nerve stimulation

Reduces chronic fatigue

The vagus nerve influences the body's behavior in certain situations. When the vagus nerve is overstimulated, it triggers a response from the sympathetic nervous system, which puts the body in a state of maximum alertness. However, constant alertness can lead to a feeling of thirst and exhaustion. Exhaustion is not just a temporary condition but rather a serious, chronic condition that can leave you feeling tired no matter what you do or how hard you work. This condition is influenced by both the health of the digestive and nervous systems and the vagus nerve.

Chronic fatigue, which can make life unpleasant, is caused by the vagus nerve. In addition, breathing problems can contribute to a condition known as false vagus tone, which is often overlooked but can significantly impact the body. Therefore, it is essential to understand the vagus nerve's role in the body and its influence on bodily functions, including breathing, to maintain optimal health.

Fights chronic inflammation

Since the vagus nerve is the primary source of communication between the body and the brain and allows feedback in both directions, it is primarily responsible for detecting inflammation in the body. The brain learns of inflammation if it can detect it at all, primarily through the detection of cytokines. It can then ensure that the appropriate amount of anti-inflammatory hormones is released. This means the inflammation is regulated appropriately - neither too strong nor too weak.

When the right response is used, people have normal levels of inflammation. Inflammation is necessary, for example, in the case of an injury or a mild infection. In some people, however, the inflammatory response is severely suppressed, resulting in immune deficiency. On the other hand, those who have too strong a reaction can have a solid inflammatory response that attacks itself.

The vagus nerve controls inflammation; when its tone is low, you will notice much more inflammation in your body. Conversely, when the nerve is stimulated, the immune system calms down. As a result, there is less chronic inflammation and better health.

Like everything else in your body, your immune system can malfunction, but it has significant side effects when it does. Chronic inflammation is detrimental to your health and, if severe enough, can even lead to death. When inflammation gets out of control, your own body can kill you. That is why autoimmune diseases kill people.

Avoiding false immune system reactions is preferable, but the current technique is giving people drugs that suppress the immune system. Unfortunately, these are the same drugs used to treat cancer, each with side effects. It is also not a good idea to suppress your immune system for a long time, as this exposes you to various other diseases and limits your lifestyle.

It is much better to use natural techniques to reduce inflammation. A healthy diet and avoiding sugar and processed foods are good, but frequent vagus nerve stimulation is also helpful. It helps your body to inhibit inflammation and prevent the formation of more white blood cells, which can be problematic if you have too many of them.

Improved sleep

Because of the relationship between the vagus nerve and the parasympathetic nerve, which controls the resting and digestive modes, inactivation of the vagus nerve can lead to sleep disturbances. Due to the increased sympathetic response, when the parasympathetic responses are dampened, the person will have difficulty sleeping well because the nerve that is supposed to regulate their ability to sleep is not controlling itself.

Vagus nerve stimulation has been used to treat epilepsy, using an implant to stimulate the vagus nerve electrically. However, it has also been found to affect regulatory capacity directly. In addition, it is associated with increased daytime alertness, meaning that the sufferer can stay awake for longer, especially if they have narcolepsy or similar. The problem, however, is that it has been found that the vagus nerve stimulator, especially the electrical stimulator, can cause an increase in apnoea. Apnoea can also increase the frequency of seizures, so it is difficult to determine whether electrical stimulation of the vagus nerve is suitable for people struggling with sleep apnoea or other sleep disorders.

Improved breathing

Our breathing is controlled by the lungs, which in turn are controlled by the vagus nerve via the neurotransmitter acetylcholine. Proper breathing is an effective way to deal with pain and manage stress by calming the body.
Relaxation techniques such as meditation and yoga also include breathing techniques, as correct breathing relaxes the body.

Improvement of memory and other cognitive disorders

Stimulation of the vagus nerve has been found to improve memory by releasing the neurotransmitter noradrenaline in the amygdala, which is part of the limbic system. This means activating the vagus nerve can help alleviate some cognitive disorders' effects.
The vagus nerve is also important for emotional and cognitive health. Vagus nerve stimulation is a common treatment for depression and drug-resistant epilepsy. Because the vagus nerve responds to traumatic events, vagus nerve stimulation is also used to treat anxiety and fear. The condition of your vagus nerve determines how likely you are to be emotionally affected long after a trauma.

Low heart rate variability is an essential indicator of increased emotional sensitivity to trauma. This is an indication that the vagus nerve is not functioning correctly. Under normal, non-traumatic conditions, one of the main functions of the vagus nerve is to reduce the heart rate. However, when the body is threatened, the ability of the vagus nerve to regulate the heart rate is reduced. This allows the sympathetic nervous system to activate defense responses, increasing heart rate. If the body's defense system is constantly activated, there is a high risk that the function of the vagus system will be damaged over time. As a result, the body's ability to adapt to stressful and potentially traumatic events suffers.

Higher heart rate variability in every day, stress-free situations is considered a sign that a person has a healthy ability to regulate emotions and cope with stress. However, when the vagus nerve runs at full speed, it shows psychological flexibility or the ability to manage emotions efficiently and adapt positively to the environment.

On the other hand, low resting heart rate variability indicates an impaired ability to regulate the emotional response to threatening, stressful events. This lower resting heart rate is often associated with increased trauma exposure and mental illness, poor physical health, aggression, anger, depression, anxiety, and PTSD. Individuals with lower resting heart rate variability are more vulnerable to stress and take longer to recover from stressful or traumatic experiences. In a study of 45 subjects with PTSD, depression, and intermittent explosive disorder, their resting heart rate variability was lower than that of 29 other subjects who did not have the above disorders.

Another function of the vagus nerve is to reduce aggressive behavior in people with ADHD (attention deficit hyperactivity disorder). However, a substance that decreased aggression no longer worked when the vagus nerve was removed in a test on a rodent model with ADHD. This suggests that in ADHD, the autonomic nervous system is disturbed, resulting in poor cardiac control. It has also been shown that cardiac vagal management is lower in ADHD children, especially in children who are not treated. This decreased cardiac vagal control reactivity is mainly observed when children with ADHD perform self-regulation and emotion-regulation tasks.

The influence of the vagus nerve on mental health could be due to the connection between the brain and the gut, the so-called gut-brain axis, as the vagus nerve is one of the most central means of communication between the two.

Weight management

The vagus nerve facilitates communication in the gut-brain axis. When the function of the vagus nerve is impaired, it loses the sensitivity that allows it to sense that the stomach is full. If the vagus nerve cannot send a message to the brain that the stomach is full, it means that you cannot know when you are full or not, which can lead to overeating. Stimulation of the vagus nerve increases its sensitivity to the stomach's satiety signal, and this increased sensitivity leads to a faster feeling of fullness and, thus, less food intake.

Stress management

We are in flight or fight mode when the sympathetic nervous system is active. The release of the stress hormone cortisol is one of the characteristics of fight or flight mode. The adrenal glands produce cortisol, a stress hormone. The sympathetic nervous system secretes cortisol in response to various stressors.

In contrast, elevated cortisol levels over time have numerous negative consequences, such as weight gain, high blood pressure, insomnia, and chronic fatigue. With its parasympathetic effects that inhibit sympathetic responses, the vagus nerve can effectively inhibit cortisol release by putting the body in a calm and relaxed state. As a result, people with a stronger vagus nerve response recover more quickly from illness or stress.

Improved moods and gut feelings

Have you ever walked down a dark alley and felt the hair on the back of your neck stand up? Or have you just met someone and had an instinctive reaction that you couldn't explain? Well, that's called a gut feeling, and although many of us think of them as whims or fads, gut feelings are actually real. The gut is able to communicate your feelings to the brain via the vagus nerve in the form of electrical impulses. This communication, facilitated by the vagus nerve via the gut-brain axis, is crucial to our mental health as it influences our behavior.

Improved immune system

The function of the vagus nerve in inhibiting inflammation is involved in the activity of the immune system. With any infection or injury, the resulting inflammation triggers sensory input conducted to the brainstem via the afferent vagus nerve. From here, efferent nerves send signals to the spleen and other organs. This activity helps with communication between immune cells, which shows how important the vagus nerve's role is for the immune system's optimal functioning.

Improved heart health

The sympathetic and vagus nerves cause a modification of the heart rate. The sympathetic nerve speeds up the heart, while the vagus nerve keeps it as slow as possible. A significantly low heart rate, especially under stress, indicates that the vagus nerve is strong and functioning correctly. A healthy vagus nerve can also help you live longer. According to some studies, a low heart rate can lead to a longer life. A healthy vagus nerve keeps the heart rate low, which means it can contribute to a longer life.

A dysfunctional heart rate is caused by the vagus nerve's inability to lower the rhythm when the body is under stress. As a result, it takes several minutes for the heart to return to its resting state. Recovery refers to returning to a resting heart rate from a high heart rate after the stressors have activated the sympathetic muscles. How long the body takes to recover is determined by the vagus nerve. A strong vagus nerve lets you calm your nerves and quickly lower your heart rate. A disturbed heart rate has the opposite effect.

In addition, the vagus nerve is overloaded, and the sympathetic nerve is underloaded. To maintain balance, the work is divided into two compartments. The parasympathetic nervous system has the task of slowing down the heart rate, while the sympathetic nervous system has the task of speeding up the heart rate. When the parasympathetic nervous system works harder than the sympathetic nervous system, the heart rate is too low due to an imbalance in the nervous system, leading to fainting and a temporary loss of consciousness. Syncope is the medical term for fainting. Fainting is not directly dangerous, but it is unpleasant. It can affect the ability to function normally. It can also be humiliating at inconvenient times in public places.

The person does not necessarily have to be ill or have a pre-existing condition. For example, syncope can occur in otherwise healthy people. It has no long-term effects and is not life-threatening, but it can devastate mood and self-confidence.

Many people believe that a sudden physical head tilt causes this imbalance. This includes movements such as standing up too quickly or sitting down after lying down for a long time - the sudden change in posture alters the direction of blood flow and the location of blood pooling. The difference is too abrupt for the heart muscles to adjust quickly. In our hypothetical scenario, the blood pooling shifts from the chest to the abdomen. This leads to a change in blood pressure, which lowers it significantly and triggers the seizure. The autonomic nerves keep the blood pressure stable, but they have failed miserably in this case. As they try to regain control, the person begins to regain consciousness. The attack exhausts the body, fatigues it, and causes nausea.

However, it does not explain why the autonomic nervous system could not function properly during the postural change. It could not properly regulate the blood vessels and the heart muscles to allow the action described above. Dysautonomia refers to a decrease in the ability of the autonomic nervous system to regulate the nerves. Dysautonomia can be a hereditary disease. Other non-hereditary diseases that can cause it are Ehlers-Danlos syndrome and Charcot-Marie-Tooth disease. Dysautonomia can also be a physical manifestation of other digestive and autoimmune problems, such as Chiari malformation, physical trauma, surgery, or pregnancy.

This could be due to a lack of nutrients needed by the components of the nervous system or an increase in toxins in the body. These facts are caused by the inability of the nerves to react quickly.

Faulty breathing can also directly affect the nerves of the autonomic system and the organs they supply. Chronic neuroinflammation, ulcerative colitis, sarcoidosis, Sjögren's syndrome, Crohn's disease, Parkinson's disease, and amyloidosis are examples of these diseases. The degree of vasovagal syncope varies from person to person. The condition can range from mild to severe. You should know that vasovagal syncope is not a disease in its own right. Rather, it is a symptom of a more significant problem. People who have fainting spells should see a doctor. Neurological tests, such as an MRI scan, are probably needed. Sometimes, however, vasovagal syncope results from an improperly functioning autonomic nervous system, particularly an overactive vagus nerve, and an underactive sympathetic nerve.

This is often the case when the body cannot accurately control blood pressure and heart rate.

The vagus nerve regulates our heart rate and acts as a natural pacemaker. It can effectively slow down our heart rate when it is too fast, as it is in stressful situations, by stimulating the heart muscles. Conversely, blood pressure rises when the heart rate is elevated, putting stress on the heart tissue and blood vessels.

The vagus nerve effectively lowers blood pressure and, thus, the pressure on the heart muscles by reducing the heart rate. A healthy vagus nerve is therefore important for cardiovascular health and the prevention of diseases such as hypertension.

In cardiovascular diseases, the regulatory function of the autonomic nervous system is disturbed. The parasympathetic and sympathetic nervous systems are two branches of the autonomic nervous system. To regulate the electromechanical function of the heart, these two branches must always be in balance. If this balance is given, the heart's cardiac output remains optimal despite various metabolic and environmental stress factors. Many heart diseases, such as chronic heart failure and hypertension, are closely related to imbalances characterized by decreased parasympathetic activity and increased sympathetic drive. Stimulation of the vagus nerve improves cardiovascular function and heart failure symptoms while normalizing autonomic function.

A significant decrease in total cholesterol, triglycerides, LDL, visceral adipose tissue, and plasma insulin was observed when obese and insulin-resistant rats were fed a high-fat diet and received vagus nerve stimulation. In addition, Vagus nerve stimulation significantly reduced blood pressure and improved heart rate variability in the subjects. It also improved the function of the left ventricle and strengthened the mitochondrial function of the heart.

Vagus nerve stimulation has also been shown in numerous studies to be helpful for stroke patients. A recombinant tissue-type plasminogen activator is used within 4.5 hours after a stroke. This can lead to rapid restoration of cerebral blood flow. This has several benefits but can also lead to an exaggerated inflammatory response that exacerbates ischaemic damage and can be extremely dangerous to the individual. In animal experiments with toxins in the blood (endotoxemia), stimulation of the vagus nerve significantly lowered systemic levels of pro-inflammatory mediators such as interleukin 1 beta (IL-1), interleukin 6 (IL-6), tumor necrosis factor-alpha (TNF-) and the DNA-binding protein high-mobility group box 1 (HMGB-1).

In the acute phase of an ischaemic stroke, stimulation of the vagus nerve also protects neurons, which can reduce infarct volume. In a study on rodents, researchers caused strokes in experimental animals by occluding their middle cerebral artery. Then, 30 minutes after the artery was blocked, the researchers performed vagus nerve stimulation. This led to a 50% reduction in infarct volume. Neurological scores also improved with this application.

In addition, stimulation of the vagus nerve was found to prevent endothelial dysfunction, often caused by high blood pressure. This was found in a test with hypertensive rats prone to strokes. In addition, stimulation of the vagus nerve was shown to prevent the stiffening of the aorta that would otherwise occur in the test animals. According to the researchers, the anti-inflammatory effect of the vagus nerve was responsible for the positive results they observed.

Fights digestive problems

The intestine or digestive tract is the area most often discussed regarding the vagus nerve. It is indeed very influential in both directions. Poor vagal tone leads to poor gut health, which can cause low vagal tone. Therefore, it is crucial to treat the body as a whole. Here are some of the diseases associated with damage to the vagus nerve in the gut:

Crohn's disease: This is an inflammatory disease of the intestinal tract. It is often painful and leads to diarrhea and weight loss. People with Crohn's disease suffer from constant malnutrition and intense pain throughout the day due to intestinal problems.

Colitis: Crohn's disease and other inflammatory bowel diseases can lead to colitis, which is inflamed intestine tissue. It can lead to ulcers in the intestinal mucosa, infections, fever, and extreme abdominal pain.

IBS (irritable bowel syndrome): IBS is an inflammatory bowel disease often associated with Crohn's disease but only affects the large intestine. Like Crohn's disease, it causes abdominal pain and intestinal discomfort.

Digestive disorders: Indigestion, which manifests itself as discomfort in the stomach after eating and occasional heartburn, is usually caused by a lack of stomach acid. This is also due to the vagus nerve not being sufficiently stimulated, which signals the stomach to produce more acid.

Interstitial cystitis: Painful urination is usually due to a bladder infection, but the pain and pressure in the bladder occur even without an infection. There is no clear cause for it. Since the vagus nerve is part of the bladder's stimulation system, influencing it can relieve this bladder problem.

Holey gut: This is a condition where the small intestine's lining is damaged and starts to let larger particles through. Instead of filtering out toxins and bacteria, it allows them to enter the blood. If the damage is extensive enough, it can even let chunks of food through. This causes the person to become very ill. One can be malnourished and tired and get sick with everything that comes along.

SIBO (small intestine bacterial overgrowth): The small intestine has a variety of bacteria, but when there is an imbalance due to antibiotics (as was the case with me), bacteria that have no business being in that area of the intestine can take up residence and get out of control. Depending on the circumstance, this can lead to pain, bloating, diarrhoea, or constipation.

The importance of the role of the vagus nerve cannot be overstated. It is also involved in many other aspects of human health. For example, when the vagus nerve is stimulated, trigeminal pain can be reduced. The vagus nerve is also thought to be involved in vagoglossopharyngeal neuralgia, a rare form of trigeminal neuralgia. In addition, stimulation of the vagus nerve has also been found to help relieve cluster headaches and migraines. In addition, stimulation of the vagus nerve can potentially prevent kidney damage, as has been found in rodent studies. The vagus nerve is also involved in the lower oesophageal sphincter, particularly in its reflex relaxation, which affects gastro-oesophageal reflux disease (GERD).
Perhaps one of the most interesting aspects of the vagus nerve's involvement in human health is that it can trigger the cough reflex. Furthermore, when the vagus nerve is stimulated, inflammatory conditions are reduced due to the anti-inflammatory properties of the nerve. According to researchers, vagus nerve stimulation may be promising in treating irritable bowel syndrome, rheumatoid arthritis, postoperative ileus, and inflammatory bowel disease.

Chapter 11: How to massage the vagus nerve

Massage has been known for some time as an effective way to improve circulation. According to research, it is one of the simplest and most sensitive techniques for improving vagal tone. The vagus nerve is stimulated by massaging certain areas of the body, such as the carotid artery. According to one study, this practice can help reduce seizures. Carotid massage, which involves applying digital pressure to the innervated carotid sinus, is an excellent method for stopping supraventricular tachycardia (SVT) caused by paroxysmal atrial tachycardia. However, Vagus nerve stimulation has recently been shown to be a superior method. In the treatment of refractory epilepsy, the vagus nerve is stimulated with a pacemaker. This method can reduce seizures and achieve therapeutic neurological results. However, this technique should not be tried at home as it can lead to fainting if not performed correctly.

In addition, pressure massage has been shown to activate the vagus nerve and promote weight gain in underweight infants. Reflexology is also helpful for improving heart rate variability (HRV) and increasing vagus activity, resulting in lower heart rate and blood pressure.

Specific massage techniques can stimulate the vagus nerve. Reflexology has been shown to stimulate the vagus nerve, improving vagal tone and reducing anxiety. Foot massages can reduce the fight or flight response and stimulate the vagus nerve, but other types of massage can also help. This is a very physical method of stimulating the vagus nerve, which can be highly effective if used correctly. After all, who doesn't appreciate a good massage?

You can receive a massage in just one area of your body or a full body massage. Allow a loved one or expert to stimulate that nerve for you. Whatever you choose, make it as relaxing and enjoyable as possible. For example, if you don't like your feet being touched, you won't benefit as much from a foot massage as if you enjoy it.

Pressure massages can stimulate the vagus nerve. These massages help babies gain weight by stimulating the intestines, primarily controlled by the vagus nerve. Foot massages can also increase the activity of the vagus nerve and, at the same time, decrease the heart rate and blood pressure, reducing the risk of heart problems.

Facial massages that involve the neck are great for stimulating the vagus nerve, but a good shoulder massage from a friend can also achieve the same results. If you need another reason to get a massage, now you have one.

A massage relaxes you immediately, and your parasympathetic instinct for rest and digestion is activated when you are relaxed. When you use your parasympathetic nervous system, you unintentionally stimulate your vagus nerve.

Massages on different body parts, especially along the carotid artery (the side of the neck where the pulse is measured) or on foot, are extremely effective for stimulating the vagus nerve. For example, one study found that massages in the neck area reduce seizures, while foot massages can help increase heart rate variability (HRV) and vagus activity while lowering heart rate and blood pressure, reducing the risk of heart disease. If you have never had a spa massage, I recommend doing so. However, if you don't have the funds, you can do it from your home. For example, have your foot massaged by your spouse, partner, or someone you trust. However, having a carotid massage done at home by a layperson is not advisable, as this may lead to fainting.

Scientific research has shown that massages stimulate and increase the activity of the vagus nerve. Therefore, some areas of the body can be massaged to achieve the desired result. One such place would be massaging the foot. This helps to relieve pressure on the nerves and increase heart variability. For this reason, many people prefer a foot massage when they are suffering from some form of exertion or stress. The areas around the neck can also be massaged to stimulate the vagus nerve. This reduces heart spasms and improves communication between the brain and the vagus nerve. It is advisable to have a massage at least once a month.

Abdominal massage is a natural anti-inflammatory method.

Fortunately, natural techniques can stimulate this nerve and improve your vagal tone to regulate the immune system better, relax the body and mind, and inhibit inflammation. Studies suggest that stimulating the vagus nerve acts as a natural anti-inflammatory and relaxing agent, reducing the production of pro-inflammatory cytokines and calming the nervous system.

A type of self-abdominal massage is a method to minimize inflammation and tone the vagus nerve. Intense pressure stimulation has been shown to activate the vagus nerve, improve digestive tract flow and performance, and boost insulin production to better control blood glucose in premature infants (adult studies pending). In addition, the combination of manual manipulation and vagus nerve stimulation can have a powerful anti-inflammatory effect.

This abdominal massage only takes a few minutes and is easy to do at home. This procedure is best done on an empty stomach a few hours after eating. Start slowly to see how the body responds. Lie down on a soft floor mat or couch.

Place your hand under your breastbone or sternum. Allow gentle, stroking downward movements - move your hand down into your abdomen. Do this movement for a few minutes, riding backward, similar to riding a bicycle, from side to side.

Then make small circular movements on your belly with your fingertips. Start massaging the sides of the abdomen and slowly work your way inwards and downwards. Gradually go deeper while applying firm and relaxed pressure. Carry out this abdominal massage for several minutes. End the session with a relaxed spinal twist on two knees (Supta Matsyendrasana) for several minutes. This restorative yoga pose aids digestion and opens the fascia and diaphragm to intensify the breath and promote an anti-inflammatory response to relaxation.

Lie on your stomach and exhale while gently pressing your bottom to the floor or bed. Inhale here for a few moments while opening your lower back. When you are ready, tense your abdominal muscles as you inhale and bend your knees towards your shoulders. As you exhale, support yourself with your hands on the surface, including your back, and stretch your arms to the side.

With a slow inhalation, lift the feet slightly higher than the knees, and then with an exhalation, slowly drop both legs to the left towards the floor. Keep the thighs up to the shoulders, the feet, and the elbows close together. Remain in this posture for 30-60 seconds. Take long, deep breaths while gently moving from side to side as you exhale. Try this simple exercise to reach the capacity of your vagus nerve. Do these methods for a few minutes, once or twice daily for several weeks. You will be amazed at how much stress it relieves, how well your digestion works, how well you detoxify, how well you relieve pain, and how well you inhibit inflammation!

Neck massage

Massaging the neck can benefit vagal tone and stimulate the vagus nerve. This is an excellent way to relieve muscle tension and improve vagal tone. It also relieves pressure on the joints that you may feel. Many people suffer from neck pain, which can be caused by stress, poor support, or insufficient sleep. This can lead to pinched nerves or tension that can quickly and easily affect vagal tone. Neck tension is generally bad for the body, but it can be disastrous for people with vagal tone problems.
So what is the simplest solution to this problem? One of the easiest methods is to take a foam roller and gently roll your neck. Also, examine your pillows. Buy new pillows or look around your home for new ones. They should not be too soft or too hard. Lift your neck slightly when you sleep to relieve any muscle tension that may be present.
Sometimes a light rubbing where the neck meets the shoulders is also an excellent way to restore vagal tone. Many like to do this; sometimes, you can feel the tension directly.

Massages for migraine

Migraines are extremely painful, and when they occur, it is easy to lose your balance no matter what you are doing. Migraines manifest differently in each person, with different triggers and pain points. The key to fighting migraines is to apply the right kind of pressure to the trigger.

These trigger points are usually located in the connective tissue between the skin and the bones. Although your migraine pattern may differ, the trigger points are generally the same. A light massage of these points can significantly relieve the pain by activating ventral circulation. Tension and hardening in these trigger points are responsible for migraine headaches.

These trigger points are located from the auricle over the neck to the trapezius muscle in the back, where it meets the back shoulder. They are on both sides of the neck and head. If you suffer from migraines or are helping someone deal with them, run your hands along this chain and feel the muscle there.

You will notice that some parts of this muscle feel firmer and harder than the rest. If you work on these points, you can significantly reduce the pain. The most important thing when massaging is to use the same technique as in the previous exercise. It would help to not press against the muscle with all your strength. Instead, gently use your fingers to reduce the tension. Hold the skin toward the greatest resistance and look for a sign indicating ventral activity.

Once you have discovered this point, go along the chain of trigger points and keep feeling for tension. Slowly but surely, you will feel relief. You can push hard against the trigger points, but this force will put the body in a dorsal state. A dorsal state also reduces pain, but without the interference of the ventral circulation, this state is not desirable.

The body needs time to regenerate from flipping over into the dorsal state. Instead, it is much better to apply light pressure and activate the ventral state so that the person can function again immediately.

Full body massage

Massages are great for your body, as we have already established in relation to your neck, but did you know that they are also good for your vagus nerve? Massaging the feet, the artery, and the area near the right side of the neck, can also help stimulate the vagus nerve. A good massage is helpful because it relieves tension and stimulates the vagus nerve.

Another good way to stimulate the vagus nerve is to massage your feet because your feet often send signals directly to your brain when you are tired, stressed, anxious, etc. When you massage your feet, you stimulate your vagus nerve, which sends signals directly to your brain. Some people don't like foot massages because they are uncomfortable. However, if you want to stimulate your vagus nerve properly, you should consider this type of massage. If tingling is a major concern for you, you can always apply more pressure to your feet. A full-body massage is also an option for those with tension throughout the body which need a deeper massage to relieve it.

By massaging the whole body, blood circulation is significantly stimulated. Blood circulation is indispensable for a healthy body. The vagus nerve is also directly connected to blood flow.

In addition to the feet and the neck, you should also massage the areas behind the ears and other parts of the face, such as the temples and cheeks. These areas also favor blood circulation.

Massages are excellent as they increase vagal modulation and improve heart rate variability, which in turn reduces sympathetic response. Also, massages feel lovely and are a great way to pamper yourself after a stressful day.

Aromatherapy

Aromatherapy is another good way to stimulate the vagus nerve. The power of scents is captivating and can trigger many memories associated with certain scents.

Happy scents are really good because they evoke a playful smell and a positive memory in you. Scents that make you feel "warm and cozy" can also help stimulate your vagus nerve.

Aromatherapy is a therapeutic method that uses essential oils from plants. It is an inexpensive, low-risk way to manage anxiety and stimulate the vagus nerve.

Many use it to relieve the symptoms of anxiety and stress. Have you ever smelled a wonderful fragrance and immediately felt happy or relaxed? That's your vagus nerve at play here.

The vagus nerve sometimes responds to scents, and the calming effect of aromatherapy directly affects the parasympathetic system and the vagus nerve. It is an enchanting feeling when you reach a relaxed state.

Lavender helps to reduce anxiety and stress and has a calming effect on the body and mind. You can use it in a diffuser, spray it on your pillows or even use a lavender essential oil and put a few drops under your tongue. This way, you can get the complete effect of the oil. I also like to use tea tree oil, lemon balm, or rosemary oil, as these oils have natural healing properties and smell fantastic.

You can use them in different ways. Using them at home in the form of a vaporizer is one of the most popular methods. Be careful if you have pets or small children, as the oils can be harmful to them. You can also apply the oils to your arm and smell them. Inhale them for a moment to absorb the properties, and then exhale.

Especially with lavender essential oils, I also like to put a few drops of them under my tongue. However, I do not recommend doing this with every single essential oil, as some of them are not healthy when ingested.

Finally, you can use aromatherapy behind the ears as a massage oil. In this case, dilute it with some carrier oil before massaging it into the ear area. This practice feels not only pleasing but also naturally stimulates the vagus nerve. Another advantage is that it smells fabulous. The massage effect combined with the smell will immediately relax and calm you.

Do you have a smell that you like and that evokes pleasant memories? Take a nice whiff of it and breathe deeply. You should feel your body relax naturally. Choose lovely fragrances that evoke pleasant memories and use them. They will do wonders for the body too.

Although aromatherapy has a bad reputation for being new-age, it has a tremendous calming effect on the autonomic nervous system, which we remember is the fight-or-flight response. Aromatherapy can help trigger calming sensations and relax the body and mind.

Don't discount aromatherapy just because it seems like a hippy practice. It is a wonderful way to naturally activate your vagus nerve and get the response you want from your body.

And not only that: aromatherapy is in a way comparable to diaphragmatic breathing. When you inhale fragrances, you stretch your diaphragm and let air flow in. As we remember, diaphragmatic breathing is an extraordinary exercise to slow the heartbeat and relieve stress and anxiety. So aromatherapy and diaphragmatic breathing are connected in some way.

Try it out for yourself. See what aromatherapy can do for you.

Chapter 12: Can a vagus nerve diet improve your health?

Nutrition and eating habits

It is no secret that healthy eating is crucial for your health and fitness. Nutrition is essential in every way - not only for your physical health but also for your mental health.

We have a strong attachment to our food. We socialize at holiday meals, socialize over food and seek refuge in comfort food when things go wrong. Yet, eating more or less than usual is one of the most common signs of depression, showing that emotions and food are very closely linked.

Nutrition means much more than eating lettuce and macadamia nuts for a slim waist and shiny hair. Unfortunately, we tend to be easily swayed away from foods that offer us the quick comfort of being particularly tasty in the modern world. We tend to forget that food is not an act of war against our bodies but an act of love.

Diet has an influence worth mentioning on how one feels and perceives life. No one says you can't eat ice cream or have dinner with your family on holidays. You just have to understand what proper balance means.

This does not refer to any fad diet. Regardless of the need to promote extremely healthy diets, the truth is that no diet prohibiting you from eating certain foods can be genuinely balanced.

The good functioning of the vagus nerve is related to everything you eat. Ensure that everything you feed your body is nutrient dense and an actual value to the body. In addition, some foods are thought to be particularly effective in maintaining a healthy nervous system. These include the following:

- Dark greens (like spinach and kale)
- Dark chocolate
- Broccoli
- Salmon and fatty fish

Research has also shown that healthy fats positively affect the vagus nerve. According to a 2005 study, good fats can reduce inflammation by stimulating the vagus nerve. Although this is not technically "activating the vagus nerve," it is one of the simplest things you can do to strengthen the function of this vital nerve in the human body (and its connection to other areas of the body) (Luyer, 2005).

Many aspects of your health can be improved just by eating right, but did you know that this also significantly impacts your vagus nerve? I wasn't aware that a healthy lifestyle had other benefits until I had already changed my eating habits, such as increased vagal tone.

It turns out that what you eat and the bacteria in your digestive tract have an impact on how your brain functions. If you take antibiotics or other medications, the bacteria in your gut can be killed or thrown out of balance. This is precisely what happened to me. So when my friend suggested I take probiotics, she was on the right track. It only takes a few bottles of kombucha to help your gut.

Here are some foods that should be included in your daily diet:

Fermented foods: Fermented foods contain healthy microbes and bacteria, so they can help restore the bacteria in your digestive tract when they are depleted. Some of the most common fermented foods are sauerkraut, cheese, kefir, kombucha, and yogurt. But you can also make fermented salsa, ketchup, and many other delicious gut-boosting foods at home.

High-fiber foods: You want to keep everything moving, and one of the signs that your gut is not healthy is constipation. So it makes sense to eat fiber, but there's another good reason for it ... Prebiotics. High-fiber foods contain prebiotics, which helps good gut bacteria thrive and reduce stress levels. High-fiber foods include everything from whole grains, seeds, fruits and vegetables, and nuts.

Calcium: Calcium is a bone-building mineral that protects the body from diseases such as diabetes and cancer. It is also essential for the proper functioning of the nervous and cardiovascular systems, including the vagus nerve. Unfortunately, calcium is one of the nutrients that the body cannot make itself, so you need to get it from food. Calcium is found in dairy products, dark green leafy vegetables such as kale or broccoli, and canned fish with softened bones.

Magnesium: Without magnesium, the heart cannot function as well as it should. This mineral is an essential part of regulating the circulatory system. It helps the heart contract properly, controls the heart rhythm, and prevents many heart problems. It is found in nuts and seeds, green leafy vegetables such as kale and spinach, figs, avocado, bananas, and seafood in general. Legumes such as beans and peas are also rich in magnesium.

Sodium: You have probably heard that salt is bad for you all your life. This is a common myth. While too much sodium is not suitable for your body, the right amount is necessary for your body to function. Wholemeal bread, cured meat, and chicken are all excellent sources of sodium. You can also use sea salt or Himalayan salt in your meals.

Potassium: Potassium: is found in all body tissues and is responsible for several functions. It helps keep the intestines moving and the muscles contracting. Potassium is also essential for nerve transmission. So it is very useful for maintaining the correct function of the vagus nerve. This mineral is found in citrus fruits, dates, spinach, beans, and melon.

Phosphorus: Calcium and phosphorus together ensure vigorous, healthy bones and teeth. Phosphorus is also helpful for energy management and keeping the vagus nerve healthy. It is also important for the regulation of hormones. Excess phosphorus is excreted through the kidneys, provided they are healthy. Phosphorus is found in chicken, eggs, cheese, tinned sardines, milk, and sunflower seeds, among other things.

Omega-3 fatty acids: Omega-3 fatty acids are valuable for brain health and can also help your digestive system. They are found in fatty fish such as salmon, flaxseed, rapeseed, soybean, nuts, and seeds. These fats help your brain and gut and boost energy, improve the immune system, and increase the efficiency of your hormone-producing glands.

Polyphenol: Polyphenols are chemicals produced by plants and processed by the bacteria in your digestive tract. They increase the number of healthy bacteria and are associated with eliminating brain fog. Polyphenols are found in green tea, coffee, olive oil, and cocoa, among others, as well as cloves, beans, nuts, soy, and berries.

Tryptophan: You probably know tryptophan as the amino acid found in turkey but also in eggs and cheese. This amino acid not only makes you sleepy on holidays, it actually converts into serotonin, the neurotransmitter responsible for feelings of happiness.

Each nutrient mentioned is important, so ensure you include them in your diet. Something must be said about eating a varied diet, so don't worry too much about it. Eat plenty of the vegetables and foods mentioned above, and you should get everything you need.

You can eat many good foods, but you should avoid a few foods. Make sure you know what these are so that you can adjust your diet accordingly.

Foods to avoid include those that promote inflammation. Refined carbohydrates, such as white bread, tend to inflame the body, as do fried foods and sodas. In fact, anything containing refined sugar can cause serious health problems, and the added inflammation boosts immune response and decreases vagal tone. If you are unsure whether a food is good for you, look at the ingredients list. You should probably leave it out if it has more ingredients than just the staples. For example, apple puree with a long list of chemicals is not the best choice and does not provide as many nutrients as puree made only from apples.

Meal planning can help you ensure your meals are rich in healthy ingredients. When preparing meals at the last minute, you are more likely to reach for what is quick and easy. You are also less likely to stock everything you need for a healthy meal. Instead, make a meal plan for the week and then shop according to the list. Planning at least a few very simple meals is a good idea. That way, you are less likely to skip something or order a takeaway.

Another way to eat healthily is to make everything in advance. Eating healthy is easy if you always have a big bowl of salad in the fridge. You'll also find that you can easily assemble a great meal with staples like beans, chicken or beef, brown rice, etc. Make sure you also have healthy snacks on hand if you are hungry. The easier you make it to eat healthily, the less likely you are to turn to fast food or processed foods that are not good for you.

A balanced diet is best for you if you focus on foods promoting gut health and avoid inflammation. The health of your gut will have a significant impact on your nervous system.

Important nutrients for the vagus nerve

Before we begin, it is important to briefly discuss the essential nutrients already mentioned - proteins, carbohydrates, fats and oils, vitamins, minerals, trace elements, and phytochemicals - and their impact on your health system. This will give you a more valuable understanding of how to drive the recovery process in reality.

Omega-3 fatty acids

These acids are extremely important for your body for various reasons. They belong to the essential minerals that the body cannot create itself. They must be obtained from external sources. Salmon, walnuts, flaxseed, soybean oil, and seaweed are the best sources of these acids. They stimulate the vagus nerve, increasing the nervous system's efficiency.

Eating foods rich in omega-3 fatty acids affects nerve impulses and gives you better control over your mental system. If you are dealing with addictions, you may not be in control because the management of your parasympathetic nervous system is weak. Foods high in omega-3 fatty acids can help bridge this gap.

Not only do they help activate the parasympathetic nervous system by increasing vagal tone and activity, but they also help eliminate bad habits and addictions. For example, suppose you see someone suffering from an addiction, such as smoking or alcohol consumption. In that case, you can recommend that they eat foods with omega-3 fatty acids, especially salmon fish.

If you eat lots of foods with omega-3 fatty acids, your body will be free of problems with high blood pressure and unbalanced heart rate. In addition, omega-3 fatty acids help prevent damage to the vagus nerve and speed up the healing process for nerve injuries.

The primary omega-3 fatty acids are eicosapentaenoic acid (EPA) and docosahexaenoic acid (DHA). Salmon, mackerel, shrimp, sea bass, oysters, and sardines are DHA- and EPA-rich fish foods, while seaweed and kelp are DHA- and EPA-rich plant foods.

Omega-3 fatty acids are essential fats our body needs but cannot produce. They are obtained from omega-3-rich foods such as salmon, walnuts, flaxseed, soybean oil, and seaweed. Fatty foods are often viewed with skepticism. But while we all need a healthy fatty diet for our mental health, the source of the fats we eat is also important. According to research, eating omega-3 fatty acids (found mainly in fish, especially fatty fish like salmon) activates the parasympathetic nervous system and increases vagal tone and activity. Therefore, we need about three times the omega-3 fatty acids to rebalance our system. Otherwise, the vagal tone of our vagus nerve decreases.

When taking eicosapentaenoic acid (EPA), an omega-3 fatty acid important for cellular functions, ensure you get enough docosahexaenoic acid (DHA) in your diet. DHA makes up about 90% of the omega-3 fatty acids in our brains. However, our bodies can only make a sparse amount of DHA from other fatty acids, so it needs to be supplied through food or supplements. So make sure you consume enough fish, oil, nuts, or seeds high in omega-3s to get high-quality DHA for your vagus nerves.

DHA and EPA are the two main types of omega-3 fatty acids. Fish diets rich in DHA and EPA are salmon, mackerel, sea bass, oysters, shrimp and sardines, while algae are plant-based diets that also contain DHA and EPA.

If you cannot meet your omega-3 fatty acid requirements with food, you may benefit from taking omega-3 supplements. You can choose from many types of omega-3 supplements rich in DHA and EPA, such as fish oil, cod liver oil, krill oil, and algae oil. I personally eat a lot of salmon supplemented with krill oil to stimulate my parasympathetic nervous system. DHA and EPA can help reduce inflammation and the risk of chronic diseases like heart disease.

Omega-3 fatty acid has been shown to help overcome addictive behaviors, reverse cognitive decline, and even help repair leaky spots in the brain. It has also been shown to increase heart rate variability in obese children, making it an important factor in various aspects of our mental health and overall well-being.

Protein

Protein contains the structural elements for the growth and recovery of body tissue and is one of the main nutrients for the healing process. In addition, protein is the primary building block for your muscles, which are your body's largest and most dynamic energy-dependent structure, accounting for 40 percent of average body weight. In contrast to its presence in muscle tissue, creatine is found in almost all body cells and tissues, including the blood.

An adequate intake of dietary protein is important for children's growth; if it is not taken in the required amount, it can lead to muscle atrophy. However, since the daily protein intake is only one gram per day, protein deficiency is uncommon in Western countries today. Nevertheless, the fear of too little protein intake is the reason for the poor dietary habits of many Western countries. This fear leads to overfilling, which can lead to obesity and be very dangerous for healing.

Many people nowadays depend on meat and animal products as convenient protein sources. Such diets are unfortunately very high in fat and do not contain fiber-free animal fats, which unnecessarily stress the digestive process. Understanding to include meat-free foods in your daily diet is a much safer and healthier way to your healing process.

Carbohydrates

Plants provide carbohydrates. Carbohydrates are the main source of fuel for the body. Starch was the old familiar name for carbohydrates, which we sometimes apply to heavier, denser carbohydrates such as squash and certain cereal flours used in bread making. Starch used to be thought of as having "empty calories," but we now know better. Marathon runners and triathletes eat a lot of pasta and rice before a big race, traditionally considered "carbohydrates" because they provide the highest total calorie output of any food. You already know these are the best high-performance long-term fuel for your bodies.

Next to potatoes, grains such as rice, wheat, oats, corn, barley, and millet are the world's most important staple foods and have long been a source of the world's greatest carbohydrate-based nutrients. These products, which contain "hard" carbohydrates, provide the fastest, most efficient, and most effective fuel for your healing process. They are high in protein, which is particularly beneficial for your gut and heart health. A diet of complex carbohydrates is also a recognized source of vitamins, minerals, trace elements, and other nutrients such as phytochemicals. To supplement, stabilize and keep your health system running smoothly and effectively, your diet should consist of about 60% complex carbohydrates.

Fats and oils

Fats and oils are central to the performance of your healing system. In particular, they promote healthy skin and nails and contribute to the structural integrity of your body's cell membranes, which help your healing system prevent infection. Fats and oils also promote the protection and insulation of nerve sheaths that improve the health of connections with your body. Your recovery system, as you know, depends on an active and accurate communication system. Often fats and oils cushion and seal the internal organs in your body, protecting them from damage and keeping the body warm. Because fats are lighter than water and contain very energy-rich nutrients, they are also a convenient way to store energy that can be used by your healing system when food intake is insufficient or scarce.

Your daily diet requires a small amount of fats and oils for this function. In contrast, fats and oils can only absorb fat-soluble vitamins and other minerals. For example, the omega-3 fatty acids contained in flaxseed oil and certain fish oils support blood clotting and can only be absorbed through fats and oils.

Certain fats and oils contain certain beneficial nutrients that have not yet been discovered. However, because fats and oils are the most compact and concentrated sources of energy in the diet, their excessive consumption contributes to obesity and other health problems, especially heart disease, which is the leading cause of death in the Western Hemisphere. Fat consumption should be limited to 10 to 25 per cent of total daily calories depending on the level of physical activity and physical health. Dr. Ornish from the University of California in San Francisco has found that a daily fat intake of 10 percent is best for supporting the healing process of heart disease. Cholesterol is a significant form of structural fat that contributes to the health and integrity of your healing process, especially your cell membranes. In addition to dietary cholesterol, your body can make its own cholesterol from other fats and oils. Nevertheless, a diet that meets the body's minimum requirements provides more cholesterol than the body needs, and when this happens, the extra cholesterol clogs the arteries, causing heart disease. Lowering net fat intake or reducing total calories while increasing daily exercise will help reduce cholesterol levels, minimize blockages, open clogged arteries, and improve blood flow in the heart.

Vitamins

Vitamins are organic substances that are necessary for the proper functioning of your healing system. They work with the body's various enzyme systems and are significant to the success of vital, life-sustaining processes that lead to healthy and weakened tissue growth, repair, and regeneration. Although vitamins are generally needed in much smaller quantities than other staple foods such as meats, fats and oils, and carbohydrates, a diet deficient in vitamins can interfere with the functioning of your healing process and contribute to disease. Vitamin requirements change over time, differ slightly between men and women, and increase during pregnancy and breastfeeding. In addition, exercise and recovery from illness and injury increase the body's need for one or many vitamins. Because of the complexity, subtlety, and largely unexplored biochemical processes and pathways in the body, more vitamins will certainly be discovered and recognized as important to our healing system in the future.

The easiest way to ensure that your healing system is adequately supplied with vitamins is to eat a healthy, balanced diet that includes plenty of whole grains, nuts, seeds, fruits, and vegetables and to limit fats and oils (certain vitamins require fat to be absorbed). However, suppose a problem occurs in a particular area of your body. In that case, you may need to supplement your normal diet with a particular nutrient or turn to foods with greater amounts of the vitamin to help the healing process.

Minerals

Minerals, as are vitamins, are also essential nutrients to support the healing process. They are needed for tissue growth, repair, and regeneration to keep the body healthy and free from disease. Minerals come directly from the earth's interior and have unique properties. The structure and function of important enzymes, hormones, and molecules, such as hemoglobin, are transported through the body. As mentioned above, almost all mineral components of the earth's core are found in small amounts in the human body. Even arsenic, which is usually considered a poison, is needed by the body in tiny amounts. Trace elements are chemically related to minerals and usually belong to the same food class. The difference between minerals and trace elements is that minerals are needed in higher quantities and their functions are better researched. We know that trace elements are necessary for good nutrition and health, but we do not know exactly what each does. Nevertheless, we know that a deficiency of trace elements in our bodies leads to impaired growth, increased susceptibility to infections, and even death. So although they are only needed in tiny quantities, trace elements are essential for the optimal functioning of your heating system.

Probiotics

Probiotics are living microorganisms (usually bacteria) found in food or supplements used to increase, maintain or improve the health of the good bacteria in our bodies, such as in our gut.

There have been sensational discoveries about the relationship between the bacteria in the gut and the vagus nerve. Research has shown that these bacteria improve brain function when the vagus nerve is stimulated. These bacteria alter the receptors that release stress hormones, depression, and anxiety. As a result, they are able to reduce the body's reaction time to stress and unnecessary worry. The vagus nerve supports the communication and flow of neurons between the gut and the brain.

When the gut microbiome is flooded with pathogenic (harmful) bacteria, the breeding ground for inflammation is created. Probiotics help the vagus nerve inhibit inflammation.

Lactobacillus rhamnosus and Bifidobacterium longum are the two main species from which most probiotic supplements are made. In addition, fermented foods such as yogurt, kefir, kimchi, sauerkraut, cheese, kombucha, and miso are also known to be rich in probiotics. Therefore, you should include these foods in your diet.

Probiotics are a group of important substances for your health and nutrition. Probiotics are produced by certain strains of bacteria that occur naturally in your intestinal tract. These strains of bacteria help your immune system fight infections, restore health and maintain proper biochemical balance in your body. More than 500 different strains of bacteria have been found to exist in your gut and help break down the food you eat, producing important metabolic by-products that are then absorbed and transported to the various cells and tissues in your body. One of these components is vitamin K, an essential component of blood clotting for the immune process. Researchers have found, for example, that eating Lactobacillus bacteria, usually known as acidophilus and found naturally in yogurt and available in commercial preparations for milk and other products, reduces diarrhea in children, reduces the risk of gut side effects when taking antibiotics, and prevents yeast infections in women. In addition, Probiotics can often fight infections, especially intestinal and respiratory infections. They can also reduce the required dose and potential risk of childhood vaccinations.

Knowing that your body is a powerful machine with an incredible healing system that requires the best energy from the purest sources is important. Repairing and restoring weakened tissue requires energy, and the energy you use in your diet greatly impacts your overall health and wellness process.

Remember to eat healthy and nutritious foods that are clean and natural and contain lots of vitamins, minerals, trace elements, fluids, and proteins. This includes most fruits, vegetables, whole grains, nuts, soups, herbal teas, juices, and wine. Ensure your diet contains enough protein, vegetables, fats, and oils. Eat natural foods representing all the rainbow colors at least once a week to get enough phytochemicals. Take the time to prepare your meals properly, eat regularly, skip unhealthy snacks, and chew your food well. To recover from a debilitating illness or disease, reduce or eliminate the meat in your diet. Refrain from eating fatty and dense foods that have no weight. Reduce your intake of alcohol and caffeine.

There are many excellent food sources. Regarding your health system diet, respect your individuality; keep your mind open and don't be too strict or fanatical about following a diet that has been successful for others but may not be suitable for you. Instead, stay informed and listen to your body as you work to meet its ever-changing nutritional needs.

The healthy bacteria in our gut stimulate positive feedback to our brain via the vagus nerve. What I'm saying is that these bacteria in our gut stimulate the release of various neurotransmitters (like serotonin, dopamine, and GABA, which are partly responsible for how we feel and what we think) in our brain, mediated by the vagus nerve. Our bodies have a lot of bacteria, both good and bad. Probiotics are live microorganisms (usually bacteria) found in foods or supplements used to increase, maintain or strengthen the health of beneficial bacteria in our bodies, such as our gut.

Lactobacillus rhamnosus and Bifidobacterium longum are the two main species from which most probiotic supplements are made. For example, research has shown that probiotics stimulate the production of important neurotransmitters that affect our mental health. Lactobacillus rhamnosus is a probiotic that improves neurotransmitter gamma-aminobutyric acid (GABA) levels in the brain. It was proven that the vagus nerve was stimulated by these probiotic bacteria, which stimulated the production of GABA. GABA has several bodily functions, including controlling anxiety and improving our mood. Bifidobacterium longum has also been shown in a clinical test to normalize anxiety-like behavior.

The vagus nerve essentially interprets the gut microbiome and initiates a response to regulate inflammation, depending on whether it detects pathogenic or non-pathogenic bacteria. For example, Probiotics help the vagus nerve fight inflammation, and when the gut microbiome is flooded with pathogenic (harmful) bacteria, the breeding ground for inflammation is created.

It is important to check your gut microbiome to know how healthy your gut is and determine if it contains enough probiotics. Probiotics in the gut microbiome can positively affect the health of your immune system and other factors.

However, always seek advice from a doctor who knows about probiotics before you start or stop taking probiotic supplements or foods.

Should you take food supplements?

It may seem that taking supplements for these essential vitamins and minerals is the better option, but is it for real?

It would help if you tried to get your nutrients from your diet as much as possible. Certain nutrients can be taken in pill form, but your body processes them best if you eat them naturally. Foods contain various nutrients that work together to help your body process them better. It is possible to replicate this, but you will find that a balanced diet is the best remedy.

If your diet is deficient in specific nutrients, supplements can be an excellent way to supplement your diet. However, try to take in everything you need through pills whenever possible.

If possible, choose food that is organically grown. This way, you can ensure that the food contains the right nutrients. Today's crops are often grown in soils high in chemicals and low in real nutrients. This does not provide as many health benefits as crops grown in naturally enriched soils with proper crop rotation. Local food is preferable because you can talk to farmers about how they grow their crops.

Change your eating style

How you eat is just as important as what you eat. Even with the best diet, you can have problems with vagal tone. Often a combination of methods is needed, and changing your eating habits is a good start.

So what does this mean? First, it would help if you took the time to observe your eating habits and find out where they are unsuitable for you. You must be mindful of your food. Don't just gobble your food without thinking or while staring at the TV. Instead, take the time to appreciate what you are eating. Smell it, look at it, and be happy that you have something good to eat.

The sensory part of eating activates the brain, the digestive system, and the vagus nerve. The food's sight, smell, and taste get everything going. Imagine smelling something delicious, and your mouth is already watering. This is just a tiny part of what happens when you are mindful of what you eat. The more attention you pay to your food, your vagus nerve becomes tense.

You should also take your time when eating and enjoy everything. This helps your body digest the food better and also increases vagal tone. If you want to ensure your tone is high, invite friends over for a meal. Sharing meals is a perfect way to strengthen the vagus nerve and automatically slows down eating as you talk and laugh together. This is an easy way to increase your vagal tone, and it's fun too.

You can eat more comfortably with others and enjoy the sights and smells, but you can also improve your eating habits by appreciating what you have. For example, be grateful when you bite into fresh fruit, and be happy that you live where you can eat well. Give thanks even for the simplest foods. They are all important; this gratitude will help improve your vagal tone.

Choose foods that you enjoy, but also healthy ones. Of course, you want to eat what is healthiest for your body, but enjoyment should also be part of the equation. So choose your food wisely and make sure you eat mindfully.

Don't expect to be able to make all these changes immediately. It has been proven that small, gradual changes bring the best results in the long term. Pick one change, e.g., more whole grains, and focus on it. Gradually, you will find it easier to get used to the changes, and you can keep making new changes.

One way to help your vagus nerve is to change your diet. Remember that your vagus nerve goes all the way to your gut. It is directly influenced by the hormone levels produced there. It can also contribute to healing and send better messages to the brain if you provide it with the nutrition it needs. This means that changing your diet can help the vagus nerve work more effectively. With a more effective nerve in place, you should be able to get results.

Mediterranean diet: You should focus on a few different diets. First, you should focus on the Mediterranean diet. This diet is highly specialized to help your body thrive by using foods that naturally inhibit inflammation. It is packed with heart and brain-healthy foods that also help to eliminate inflammation in the body. This is the perfect support you can give your body when trying to support the vagus nerve with your diet.

Fermentation: You should also focus on fermented foods when adjusting your diet. While these can take some getting used to over time, you will find that they are much more beneficial. They support the probiotics in your gut that help your vagus nerve to thrive.
High-fiber foods: Finally, you should also eat high-fiber foods. These foods act as so-called prebiotics - the probiotics in your body thrive best on fiber that you would otherwise not be able to digest. Eating fiber-rich foods gives these probiotics a wonderful feast that keeps them healthy and is responsible for giving you a healthier body at the end of the day.

Chapter 13: Most common traumas of the vagus nerve

This chapter has important implications for how we understand trauma and its consequences. I have already mentioned that the absence of a combat response is not a sufficiently sound principle to draw conclusions from and is even harmful because the victim has no choice in this response. The dorsal system also explains how trauma victims process their experiences.

Some victims forget the experience or cannot remember it with full clarity. This is simply because their brain erases anything painful, or they cannot handle a fight or flight response. As a result, the dorsal state is activated, and the victim simply forgets or gives up ultimately.

In addition, it is important to remember that current stimuli and past experiences influence the nervous system's response. These experiences exist in our subconscious, and we are unaware of how they influence us. More importantly, the doctors treating us need to consider these past experiences.

The current trigger puts our nervous system in the same state as the previous experience. In other words: If something in your recent experience reminds you of something that happened to you, you will react the same way as you did then.

Therefore, the key to treating a victim is to realize that reactions do not happen of their own free will. People do not "give up"; they just do what their nervous system tells them to do. Consequently, they have no choice but to comply. Therefore, blaming the victim or wishing they could have done something differently makes no sense.

Since the poly vagus theory and the healing effect of the vagus nerve are still being researched in depth, there is still a long way to go before this theory is generally accepted. However, if you already use the methods to stimulate the vagus nerve, you are at the forefront of innovative science.

Trauma and neuroception

Trauma plays a central role in the way we perceive things. People who suffer from conditions like PTSD find it difficult to categorize things as non-threatening and face significant challenges in dealing with their triggers. One of the reasons why trauma is particularly challenging is because of the way the brain learns and processes information.

The brain consists of many cells, called neurons, which are connected and form a so-called neural network (Oschman, 2016). Together, these networks form a body of information. When sensory input is perceived, the connections are activated, creating a sensation. The corresponding ANS pathway is activated to maintain homeostasis in the perceived environment.

The biggest weakness in all of this is neuroception. This is the filter through which we view the world, and as we have seen, it is very easily manipulated. Profound emotional experiences, whether positive or negative, can distort neuro perception to the point where we turn facts upside down and become blind to everything else.

One example is the level of political debate. Contrary to popular belief, political debate has never had a high level. One reason is people need to stick to their perception (neuroception) no matter what. Social media is a vast confirmation machine that only shows us what we want to see, leading to our prejudices becoming entrenched and reinforcing existing neural networks.

The brain is predisposed to minimize the effort required to make a decision. That is the goal of learning. When you sit down to drive your car, you don't want your brain to go through the whole learning process again. Otherwise, you would never get anywhere. While this learning and reduction of effort are particularly helpful when driving, brushing your teeth, cooking, etc., it is actively harmful when it comes to neuro perception colored by trauma.

Your brain reacts the way it has always responded, and if you try to question this existing behavior, it simply rebels. So why should you do anything differently? Remember that learning new things involves effort, which is also why we learn much less than children as we age. We just don't feel like making an effort.

It is much easier to cling to what we already know and stick to it even when we know it is wrong or not based on fact because the alternative is just too much work. So what is the point of this whole discussion? Well, first of all, changing habits and beliefs requires using an equal and opposite force.

In other words, you need to perform new behaviors and new ways of thinking with a high level of positive emotion (why would you deliberately expose yourself to negative emotion?) and then repeat this action repeatedly. This is how learning takes place. With the exercises presented in the previous chapters, you can simplify the learning process for yourself as you adjust to new ways of thinking and improve your life.

All in all, the Polyvagal Theory helps you to become more aware of what state of mind you are in. This awareness alone is powerful enough to get you out of your current state of mind and into another. Of course, I'm not saying you should expect miracles, but is change possible? Yes, it definitely is!

Trauma, PTSD and the Vagus Nerve

Although no one wishes for trauma, it is something that almost all of us might experience at some point in our lives. We are all exposed to trauma through an event that happens to us, whether it is the loss of a loved one, an accident, or being the victim of a crime. Trauma knows no boundaries. It does not differentiate between people.

However, they have a direct and significant impact on the brain. The vagus nerve is the great regulator of these traumatic experiences, and how the vagus nerve deals with the situation can have very different effects on your behavior. Your vagus nerve has done a great job of mitigating the long-term effects of stress - great! You will most likely recover from your trauma without any lasting effects.

However, if you are not careful, you may encounter additional difficulties. Other problems can occur if your vagus nerve is not functioning normally or if your vagus nerve has difficulty keeping up with what is happening in your own body. There may be a problem where you cannot deal with your feelings correctly. You will find that you are unable to deal with the stressors in your life, which can lead to post-traumatic stress disorder.

PTSD is thus a manifestation of the vagus nerve, which is never completely switched off. Normally, the mind can calm down after a stressful event. The mind can start to slow down and relax in some way.

However, it is thought that when PTSD occurs, the body has never activated the parasympathetic state that the vagus nerve is responsible for promoting. Without the relaxation response, the body suffers as if still trapped in the traumatic experience. Memory distortions and disturbances occur. Emotions are still volatile. Anything can upset the person.

However, getting out of this state with exemplary effort is possible. To alleviate the anxiety associated with PTSD, it is necessary to be able to reactivate the vagus nerve. Only then can one concentrate on getting one's life back on track. Only when one returns to parasympathetic normality can one start living life again. When stressed, the vagus nerve has three options: Fight, Flight, or Freeze. Each of these modes has a range of manifestations. They all seem to be very distinct from each other, regardless of how you perceive them in your current life. Your conscious mind has little influence on how your body reacts to stressors and traumas; it simply responds independently.

Imagine a cat and a mouse to understand better how this works. The cat chases the mouse. When the mouse sees the cat running away, it has two choices: fight the cat or flee from it. Since mice are not known for being vicious or ferocious, nor do they have the physical equipment to fight a cat, the mouse chooses to flee. The vagus nerve is activated, creating the feeling of flight, so the mouse flees without thinking.

However, imagine that the cat now catches the mouse. It has a paw on the mouse's tail, and it wriggles and squirms to escape. Perhaps it now bites because it is trapped and has no other option. Since it can no longer escape, it fights back - or at least tries to.

When the cat puts a paw on the mouse, holds it, and catches it, the mouse suddenly stops moving. It is not dead, but it no longer struggles or wriggles. The mouse freezes.

Each of these reactions can be easily switched. For example, you can quickly switch from fight to flight to freeze and back again. However, when you are in a stress reaction, you cannot stop it and relax again. This is because your vagus nerve must be activated before you can return to the hormone level before the stress reaction, which can take 10 minutes to hours.

Each of these reactions to trauma has its own very important purpose of keeping in mind:

Fighting is what you feel when you feel threatened and think you have a serious chance of fighting off the enemy to have the best chance of survival. Your body thinks that if you fight, there must be a chance of survival.
Flight occurs when you do not believe you can fight off the threat. Your body thinks the best response is to run away rather than try to engage in a fight that could only make the situation worse.

Rigidity occurs when the body or mind sees no natural, legitimate way to survive what has happened. So instead of trying to resist or flee, the body simply freezes. It shuts down completely to at least resist the pain and suffering that would otherwise accompany it.

Vagus nerve-related treatment of trauma

The body shows other disturbing signs of post-traumatic stress - a tightness in the stomach, a sinking feeling in the stomach, a familiar pain in the mouth, or a constant sense of tiredness. So today, we know that we need to turn to the body as part of the recovery process. As a result, meditation, mindfulness, Tai Chi, Qigong, Feldink Circle, massage, craniosacral, nutritional therapy, and acupuncture are increasingly used for post-traumatic stress disorder.
Such mind-body treatments help us be less passive, aggressive, and impulsive in response to stress. As a result, our understanding of the opportunities we need to stay grounded and relaxed grows. We feel like we need this more. One way that mental-body treatments work is by activating the vagus nerve. Awareness of how this nerve works provides a deep understanding of traumatic stress and enhances our healing ability. The vagus nerve has therefore become the focus of trauma treatment.

"Mind-body treatments" work on the vagus nerve to help you regain balance. In this article, you will find a series of breathing and movement exercises designed to relax and reset the vagus nerve. Through a cycle of self-study and conscious body awareness, you will continue to develop methods to help you regain a sense of well-being and recover from trauma. The use of mind-body therapy is associated with a variety of changes in well-being, including Improving physical and mental well-being. They enable us to focus on our feelings, impulses, and behavioral motivations. This observational ability tends to improve tolerance to discomfort, which can help reduce emotional reactivity, anxiety, panic, chronic pain, and depression. In addition, mind-body treatments improve self-understanding and the ability to perceive the other person's point of view with understanding.

In addition, mental-physical treatments are promising because they require structural improvements in the autonomic nervous system, which are determined by improving the activity of the vagus nerve. The vagus nerve runs from the brain stem down through the muscles of the nose, inner ear, chest, back, lungs, stomach, and intestines. Mind-body treatments change how we relate to the world around us, encouraging us to look gently and allowing us to try new breathing or activity patterns that communicate specifically with other body parts. Another technique researchers use to calculate changes in the vagus nerve is often called respiratory sinus arrhythmia, using heart rate variability (HRV). HRV refers to the rhythmic heart rate fluctuations that occur with breathing. It is a function of the intervals between beats of the heart. Higher heart rate variability is associated with a better ability to withstand or recover from stress, while lower heart rate variability is associated with stress and anxiety. Therefore, you should consider any form of mind-body therapy that improves heart rate variability as strengthening the autonomic nervous system. As a result, the shift between emotions of anticipation and ease is smoother.

When we sense a threat (real or perceived), we change our breathing. We can get a good picture of this by looking at the reaction of animals. In certain situations, an animal may breathe rapidly into the upper chest, a protective reaction of the nervous system that enables it to run or fight in a dangerous environment. In other situations, an animal may freeze by breathing shallowly or holding its breath to avoid being detected by a predator. This reflex causes the animal to stand completely still and is a reaction to the threat of immobilization. Finally, animals are weak in certain situations, and a predator that is not a scavenger may lose interest in a dead animal. An evolutionarily older vagus nerve axis supports both the torpor reflex and the sluggish response as a member of the parasympathetic nervous system.

Above all, an animal can activate the stress reflex through breathing to maintain homeostasis until the danger is over. Nevertheless, humans also live for long periods in either highly activated (fight and flight) or weakly activated (freeze and faint) responses. This seems to be the case when the abuse is persistent and long-lasting, as in the case of complex PTSD. Indeed, we often lack the resources to process difficult or painful experiences. This can lead to physical stress and restricted breathing habits that form the basis of our posture, our way of being active, and our general sense of self.

The vagus nerve and trauma therapy

The autonomic nervous system is divided into three parts, according to Dr. Stephen Porge's polyvagal theory: the dorsal vagal system, the sympathetic nervous system, and the ventral vagal system. The dorsal vagal system is the youngest system of the parasympathetic nervous system. The dorsal vagal nerve immobilizes the body in life-threatening situations by generating a shutdown reflex. In response to a threat, the sympathetic nervous system, a relatively recent development, mobilizes the body by activating the fight-or-flight reflex. This "social interaction" mechanism is a division of the parasympathetic nervous system that allows you to calm down and communicate with others while feeling healthy.

You will learn exercises that help repair the vagus nerve; however, not all activities suit everyone. Alternatively, I encourage you to experiment with and try different breathing and action methods until you find what works best for you. Through a cycle of self-study and conscious body awareness, you will begin to develop techniques to help you maintain a sense of safety and recover from trauma. Here are a few resources to help you start: Listen to your instincts: Arielle Schwartz, Ph.D. Somatic Experiencing.

You can also improve vagus nerve health by maintaining a healthy digestive system. The "microbiome" that lives in the gut forms the internal nervous system, also known as the gut-brain. Hundreds of healthy and bacterial organisms live in the intestinal tracts in this habitat. An imbalance in your gut can cause an inflammatory response from your immune system, leading to debilitating symptoms such as anxiety and depression. You create a balanced microbiota by reducing sugar intake and identifying latent food intolerances. Finding out the causes of a gut deficiency may require the help of a doctor or nutritionist; the effort you make to incorporate these changes into your life will be worth it.

Conclusion

Thank you for staying until the end of this book, it should have been informative and valuable to you. This manuscript should be a guide to help you learn about the vagus nerve, recognize problems that can occur when the vagus nerve is not functioning correctly, and how best to deal with the discomfort caused by vagus nerve dysfunction. We hope that you have found some enlightening, helpful and practical information for you in reading this book.

As you have experienced, the vagus nerve has been debated for centuries. The truth is that we have everything we need to live a happy and fulfilled life. Unfortunately, as science has progressed, we've lost the balance between trusting ourselves and looking to the outside world for answers.

The problem is that we need a balance between ventral and dorsal activity for our lives to run without problems. If ventral activity is absent, our default states are either the sympathetic nervous system, which is the fight or flight response, or the dorsal circuit, which causes us to withdraw from life in general. Depression is a symptom of dorsal activity in the absence of ventral intervention. Anxiety is simply the sympathetic nervous system acting out its nightmares.

Your lifestyle has a significant impact on all of this. You can do all the exercise you want, but it won't do any good if you don't change your lifestyle for the better. How much you exercise, how well you eat, and how much you limit your consumption of substances that are detrimental to your long-term health influence your ventral circulation. I advise you to seek professional help immediately if vagal nerve stimulation does not work for you or you can no longer bear the burden of depression. If you share the burden with a licensed professional, you will make much faster progress and see results sooner than if you suffer in silence alone.

Incredibly, a single nervous system can control so much. Although some aspects of the vagus nerve and its activities have not yet been explored, it is clear that it is the leader of the parasympathetic nervous system. This nervous system is supposed to control the relaxation responses of the human body.

Knowing and understanding what the vagus nerve is good for can help others improve their health. Unfortunately, most people are unaware of the power of their vagus nerve and how a vagus nerve that is out of sync with the rest of the body can harm it.

The best thing is to sit down and read the whole book to find out what works for you and what does not. Then, once you have figured it out, be consistent with your exercises. The more consistent you are, the more your body will get used to the changes and experience the many benefits.

I strongly recommend that you pay attention to your vagus nerve. Even though it seems to be just another nerve in the body, it is responsible for many problems. Understand what your vagus nerve does for you and look for ways to stimulate it more.

This information helps your brain convince itself that the vagus nerve can heal you and that all treatment options make medical sense. All you have to do is act and remember that you are valuable. If you want to take control of your vagus nerve, you can start with some of the techniques described in this book. Thank you for embarking on this journey; I wish you much happiness and peace!

Made in the USA
Las Vegas, NV
08 February 2024

85460103R00089